MORE HEALING FOODS

MORE HEALING FOODS

OVER 100 DELICIOUS RECIPES TO INSPIRE HEALTH AND WELLBEING

Jane Sen

Thorsons

Thorsons

An Imprint of HarperCollins*Publishers*

77–85 Fulham Palace Road

Hammersmith, London W6 8JB

The Thorsons website address is:

www.thorsons.com

First published 2001

10 9 8 7 6 5 4 3 2

© Jane Sen 2001

Jane Sen asserts the moral right to be

identified as the author of this work

A catalogue record of this book is

available from the British Library

ISBN 0 00 711834 1

Photography by Phil Wilkins

Printed and bound in Great Britain by

Scotprint, Haddington, East Lothian

CONTENTS

Both my parents are outstanding cooks and without their delight in food and sociability I would not have discovered the fun of cooking and sharing even the most simple of meals with those you love.

INTRODUCTION

In my heart and soul I am a cook with a passion for food and an insatiable curiosity for the way the Earth produces it.

My priorities in choosing health-giving recipes for this book have been firstly that they must taste delicious – our food should nourish us but not be separate from the absolute joy of living – and secondly that they are easy to produce in the modern world. It would be wonderful if we were all able to pop out into our gardens and gather fresh ingredients for lunch, but the reality is more often a quick dash round the supermarket on the way home from work or the school run. In the course of my work, particularly at the Bristol Cancer Help Centre, people often say that they 'just don't have the time to eat well'. The recipes in this book are simple and straightforward. It may be that they take a bit longer than popping out for fast food (although considering the traffic, I even doubt that), but they don't take any longer than cooking ever did. There is no food faster than raw food and the daily inclusion of a large bowl of fresh salad will make a big difference to your health. I cannot deny that once you begin to lessen the harmful fats, sugars and salt it is sometimes the most precious ingredient of sweet time itself that will make the delicious difference in flavour. We all need to make some time in our lives to live and be well – ultimately a lot more fun than taking time out to be critically ill.

One in three people in the developed world is predicted to get cancer. We now know some of the causes of cancer: genetic dispositions, stress, infection, environmental factors, smoking, obesity, lifestyle and diet are all well researched. Often a combination of factors at a stressful period of our lives can be the trigger. Most of these causes are beyond our control, but the way we eat can always be in our control – and it's a wonderful way to change the odds in our favour.

There is a growing understanding of the truth that 'we are what we eat' and, in fact, the real truth is that we are the difference between what we swallow and what we expel. We are what is left over when our bodies have sorted, digested, absorbed and eliminated. We are entirely built of what remains. We cannot create a healthy body from anything other than good food combined with light and oxygen. Nutritional deficiency has played a huge part in the history of disease all over the world, but now it is the reverse, and we are battling with the diseases caused by dietary excess and imbalance. Our bodies are now having to deal with exposure to new levels of toxins from modern agricultural and manufacturing methods while often gaining less nutrients from foods grown at spectacular speed, stored and transported, refined and processed. The phrase 'overfed and undernourished' really does seem to describe our pattern of eating in the fast and modern world.

When we look at the vast amount of research we now have on the way our diet affects our health, we find good evidence for change. Our food can play a leading role in the prevention, management and recovery from so many things – coronary disease, strokes, high blood pressure, diabetes, asthma, eczema, cancer, urinary problems, circulatory problems, fatigue, arthritis, digestive disorders, nervous problems and stress, reproductive disorders, skin conditions, high-risk weight imbalance and infection.

Much of the ancient wisdom and many instinctive remedies of old are now being given new credibility and support from scientific evidence. The nature of research into diet and health often means that evidence can be conflicting and the sheer volume of it makes it confusing, but the worst thing is that it is not very relevant to the practicalities of everyday life – cooking, shopping and eating. Certainly something that is clear is that there is no such thing as a bad or a good food, but there are definitely bad and good diets.

I have cooked professionally now for over 26 years and for the last ten I have worked with people wishing to use their diets to help their recovery from, or to prevent, illness. Consequently, the study and research have filled almost as much of my time as talking about it and cooking. Amongst the mass of convincing evidence there are some overriding truths; rare meeting places where scientists agree. It is those places of unanimous agreement which inform the approach I recommend here.

OUR DIETS SHOULD BE HIGH IN PLANT FOODS

This is not the same as saying that everything else makes you ill. Nor does it mean that you will have a lifetime of raw carrots, although there is no doubt of the major benefits to be had from increasing the amount of raw food we eat. It means that for health and recovery we should make sure that the majority of the food we eat started out with its roots in the soil. When we remember that the word 'vegetable' in our language comes from the Latin word *vegetare*, meaning 'to enliven, to animate', we see another example of how scientific evidence is following far behind ancient knowledge. Plants contain a fantastic armoury of protective phytochemicals, and we need a lot of them all the time to keep our immune system fighting and to keep our energy levels high. A large proportion of these phytochemicals can be gained by keeping up our intake of fresh fruit and vegetables, but wholegrain bread, pasta, grains and pulses (legumes) are all part of the plant armoury too.

This book will show you many ways of getting these foods into your diet enjoyably and I hope it will give you the confidence to try new ways of your own. The only way we can truly eat for health is to really enjoy what we eat. The key is to find dishes that fit into our lifestyle and are easy to prepare. The way to eat more foods that heal and protect is to find ways of preparing them that you love. It may be that some ways of cooking retain more of some nutrients, but cooking in a variety of exciting ways is more likely to keep you eating these foods than just knowing they are good for you.

OUR DIETS SHOULD BE LOW IN ANIMAL PROTEINS

There are no recipes for dishes in this book that contain any animal products. Some people have chosen a vegan diet on the basis of personal principles or environmental factors. I have not included animal products on the basis of current evidence concerning the over-consumption of these foods and the negative effects on our health.

In general there is no doubt that meat, fish, eggs and dairy produce should be minimized when eating for optimum health. For example, it is well documented that the over-consumption of high-protein foods can reduce our ability to retain the calcium that is so necessary to protect us from osteoporosis. If you have not decided to completely avoid animal proteins, then try to start using them as a condiment or flavouring in addition to your plant-based diet rather than as a major part of a meal. Using more soya products and replacing dairy foods not only avoids saturated fats and possible digestive-intolerance reactions, but it also adds an invaluable range of phytonutrients.

One of the major obstacles that people face when they begin to consider a new way of eating is the pattern of food on the plate. In our culture and society we are accustomed to featuring the protein part of the meal and then putting something next to it – we say meat and veg, fish and chips, omelette and salad. While we design our meals in this way we undoubtedly overload ourselves with protein, which our bodies then have to store as fat. Protein is difficult and complex for our systems to process, and it consumes energy that would be much better used in support of our immune function.

Meals need to look different. We should start to let go of this 'pattern on the plate' to realize that our food is going to really feed us, then it can be in a pretty pile, in four little bowls, in a frosted glass of frothing strawberry juice, or in our pocket while we are shopping or going for a walk. Freeing ourselves of the 'slab of protein' approach opens up a whole new world of wonderful food.

OUR DIETS SHOULD BE LOW IN SATURATED FATS

We need fat to live, but excess fat in the diet can lead to a myriad of health problems. Fat comes in three basic varieties: saturated, polyunsaturated and monounsaturated. It makes sense to obtain the fats essential for health from the sources that give us the most but are the least damaging.

Saturated fats are definitely the bad guys and these are the fats that science recommends we avoid. Saturated fats are found primarily in foods of animal origin (there are some plant sources of saturated fats such as coconuts, but in general these do not behave in quite the same way in the body and they do have some health benefits). The fastest way to get potentially damaging saturated fats out of your diet is to avoid eating meat and dairy produce. Sadly, much of the refined and processed foods that we have become so accustomed to also contains an unacceptably large amount of hidden fats. So, in general, sticking to whole foods and fresh food will keep your fat intake healthy.

HIGH IN COMPLEX CARBOHYDRATES

The strange thing about carbohydrates is that when they are complex they are simple. Carbohydrates are the most available source of energy in our food and complex carbohydrates come joined to the nutrients needed in order for us to be able to digest them and gain this energy. A large proportion of any well-balanced meal should be formed of these foods, they should cover quite a lot of the plate.

Carbohydrates come in two forms: complex (eat lots) and refined (avoid). You will gain complex carbohydrates from starchy foods that are 'whole foods', ie foods that have not had much done to them before they reach you. Foods such as whole grains, brown rice and barley, wholemeal (wholewheat) flour products, beans and lentils and, of course, all fresh vegetables. The refined carbohydrates to keep to a minimum are products that use only white flour such as white bread, white pasta and commercially produced cakes, cookies, pies and pizzas, white rice, sugar and products containing sugar. There still seems to be a lot of confusion about sugar. Sugar is refined if it is in the form of a crystal, so this is definitely one area where just because it's brown doesn't mean it is healthy. My recipes will show you ways of getting these wonderful energy foods into your life and how to have sweet goodies when you want them without using refined sugar.

LOWER SALT

It seems there is no actual recommended daily amount of salt (sodium chloride), but it is certain that the usual intake far exceeds our bodies' needs. Salt intake has an enormous influence on the dynamic balance of all our cell membranes and therefore can interfere with our ability to absorb nutrients and eliminate toxins. Of course, we need sodium chloride for our cells to function efficiently, but it is naturally present in almost all fruits and vegetables. It is the sprinkling in of the white crystals when we cook or the addition of salt at the table that pushes our intake into the danger area. There is good epidemiological research into the connection between high salt intake and certain cancers, and most people will be aware of the recommendation to keep salt low to avoid and manage high blood pressure, hypertension and heart disease. This is another area where avoiding processed and refined foods will help – they are often absolutely packed with salt and the real content is not always clear on the label. Even unlikely packaged foods, like breakfast cereals, can contain large amounts. I have not included any salt in my recipes, although they certainly do contain sodium. Within the fresh ingredients this comes twinned with vital potassium which works with it to keep your cells healthy. I have aimed for rich, good flavours without the addition of salt, and I have used some ingredients such as tamari soy sauce that add a savoury flavour without containing salt in its concentrated crystal form. Not everyone has the same sensitivity to salt within the body or on their tastebuds, so bearing the recommendations in mind, I leave you to make your own choice when cooking. If you do choose to add salt, it is well worth using one of the substitutes that are high in potassium and low in sodium.

I do not intend this book to be a means of persuasion through exposing you to pages of scientific evidence – I imagine that if you have got as far as looking at recipes you are already convinced by the theory anyway. No-one has ever made their way towards good health just by reading the research – application is the key, and the recipes in this book are ways of bringing the research into the reality of really enjoyable meals. Try to stick to the guidelines and don't panic over those moments in life when it's just not possible – it's what you do most of the time that will make the big difference.

Really enjoying your food is, in itself, a major part of your nutrition. There is even scientific evidence to show how our digestive systems work better when we eat in a relaxed and happy way. You only have to have suffered from indigestion after grabbing fast food on the run to have proved this fact all by yourself. Slow down a bit around food. Digestion begins in the mouth, chewing is part of the digestive process – it can save a lot of wear and tear on your digestive tract and help you better utilize the nutrients contained in the food. It may seem strange, but it is also helpful if you look at your food as you eat it – value its colour and aroma as well as its taste and texture, and let yourself be receptive to this new energy entering your body.

The huge health benefits offered by food are gained not only from the nutrients but also from the value we give to choosing the best and freshest of ingredients. It is not important for the raw ingredients to be lavish – even the most humble of everyday foods can offer the finest culinary results, a fact exemplified by family dishes and simple country food from the Mediterranean to the Far East. Choose food that is as fresh as you can get – subtle flavours often come from volatile oils, essential fatty acids and the vitamins and minerals themselves, all of which are susceptible to deterioration once the plant is harvested. If you think of plant foods as a bit like batteries, storing energy from the sun and the earth, then once they are removed from their source of energy they fade ever after. The fresher they are, the more they give us, both in terms of nutrition and flavour.

Once you have got your fresh whole food home, it shouldn't require any special equipment or techniques to turn it into delicious dishes. To retain the most nutrients in fresh foods, keep them cool and dark in the fridge. All nuts and oils will stay fresher in the fridge too. Cooking will be a lot more fun if you make sure you have:

- *Very sharp knives.*
- *A swivel-head type of vegetable peeler (if you do peel, it will be thinner and with less waste using one of these inexpensive little tools).*

- *Some 'user-friendly' pans – heavy with good, tight lids. A light thin pan can really bring disappointing results and good ones are an investment in the pleasure of life.*
- *An electric goblet–type blender. I use one for soups, sauces and dressings.*
- *A hand blender can be very useful and easy to wash up.*
- *An electric food processor. Choose one with a metal blade, a plastic blade, a grating attachment and, if you are really lucky, a julienne slicer (this will cut raw fruits and vegetables into perfect, attractive little matchsticks).*
- *An electric juicer – choose one easy to dismantle and wash.*

I have aimed for my recipes to be enough for a main dish for four hungry people, or six as a first course or side dish. With some of the recipes that require a bit more time and effort it is often worth cooking extra and freezing some. The cooking extra and freezing trick is almost always worth it when you are cooking beans. Freeze them in small portions and you will end up with a nice variety, ready to go, for those days when you are short of time or just feeling like a bit of spontaneous creativity in the kitchen.

Last but not least, always try to read a recipe through twice before you begin.

INDEX OF RECIPES

BURIED TREASURES

DARLING BUDS

FOREST FLOOR AND SEABED

LIVE LEAVES

NO GRAIN ... NO GAIN

MEDITERRANEAN MARVELS

ROARING RAW POWER

SQUASH FOR ALL SEASONS

THIS BUSINESS OF BEANS

SWEET AND UNREFINED LIFE

BIG BULBS AND SHORT SHOOTS

Don't panic, I am not about to ask you to go out and start digging up the daffodils and tulips. I just want to honour, for a moment, the bulbs that already feature in a big way in our diets.

The mighty onion family, with more than 300 members, could provide a fascinating book of recipes on its own merits. The entire group is bursting with therapeutic compounds that are renowned for their beneficial effects on an impressive range of ailments, including bronchitis, asthma, gout, arthritis, rheumatism and urinary infections. Perhaps the most widely researched aspect of onions has been into their protective and healing properties on the blood and circulatory system. Lowering fat levels and increasing the high-density lipoproteins has a very positive effect, protecting us from all cardiovascular diseases.

The inclusion of onions in the diet has shown a measurable improvement on cholesterol levels. Garlic is a bulb with similar pharmacological benefits, so you will find that I have used this fantastic family liberally in my recipes throughout this book. Whether red, spring (scallions), pickled, raw or cooked, eating more of the onion family can only do good. Bulbs are the fleshy, fattened leaf bases that provide all the stored energy to feed the growing plant – and they will generously provide it for us too. Apart from onions and garlic, other edible bulbs are Florence fennel, leeks – which are just rather elongated bulbs – and celeriac (celery root).

Short shoots, the very beginning – the sprout of a plant – provide a wealth of enzymes and beneficial nutrients. They are live, pure foods and some of the freshest you can possibly eat, literally bursting with the potential for life. As the seeds become ready to grow, most of the nutrients are massively increased – protein by 15–30 percent. They are filled with many of the B vitamins, vitamin C, betacarotene, vitamins E and K, calcium, phosphorus and, if you let them 'green up', chlorophyll.

Almost any seed is edible once sprouted, but some are better than others and lots are now widely available to buy ready sprouted in little bags. Even the least adventurous among us may have eaten cress, snipped from little supermarket cartons, unaware of its wonderful health-giving properties.

Whole lentils, chick peas (garbanzo beans), mung beans and alfalfa are the stars for home sprouting. I find organic are much more reliable sprouters, just check them over for broken bits and pieces. Start with a handful in a large glass jar, rinse well, soak for a few hours, drain away the water and cover with a clean cloth held in place with elastic or string (I use a disposable dish cloth). Leave the jar somewhere in the kitchen that is not too hot or bright where you will remember to rinse the seeds in fresh water and drain twice daily. Most will only take a day or two to get going and will be delicious to eat any time until the point where they have developed two leaves – as long as you keep rinsing. Wash them well in a bowl of running water before using and any loose skins will float off. If you have done too many and cannot eat them fast enough you can slow them down in the fridge. Mixing a few radish seeds into them makes a pink and pretty zesty variation.

As with the familiar supermarket mustard and cress, some seeds do better in a little soil, so try soaked sunflower, wheat grain or melon seeds spread evenly on a tray of light potting compost, water well and cover with dark plastic or a cloth. Leave in a dark place, not too cold or draughty. When they sprout, uncover them and leave in the light, spraying them occasionally to stop them drying out. Once they have grown tall and are showing green leaf, harvest by snipping with scissors and throw into salads or sandwiches. Use clean potting compost (soil) each time.

They are all a fantastic, inexpensive source of very fresh food all year round. Eat some at least twice a week.

SPROUTED SALAD WITH A CITRUS DRESSING

1 whole small orange, chopped and seeds removed
1 whole lemon, chopped and seeds removed
2 teaspoons Dijon mustard
2 teaspoons tamari soy sauce – optional
pinch of ground black pepper
1 tablespoon olive oil
2 teaspoons cider vinegar

Whizz in a blender or food processor until completely smooth. You may need to add a little water or orange juice.

350g (12oz/2 cups) sprouted chick peas (garbanzo beans), well rinsed and drained
350g (12oz/heaping 2 cups) seedless grapes, cut in half
50g (2oz/scant ½ cup) sunflower seeds, lightly toasted in a dry pan
handful of fresh parsley leaves, roughly chopped
a few chopped fresh fennel or dill fronds – optional

Combine gently with the dressing.

ALFALFA AND AVOCADO WITH SESAME MAYO

85g (3oz/scant ¾ cup) sesame seeds, roasted in a
   dry pan for 5 minutes
100g (4oz/1 cup) unblanched almonds
4 tablespoons (¼ cup) olive oil
1 teaspoon Dijon mustard
juice of 1 lemon
1 tablespoon cider vinegar
2 teaspoons tamari soy sauce – optional
pinch of ground black pepper
3 tablespoons water

Reserve a spoonful of the sesame seeds and put everything else into a blender or food processor. Whizz on full power until you have 'mayonnaise'. You may need to add a little extra water or lemon juice.

2 perfect avocados – ½ per person
100g (4oz/scant 1 cup) alfalfa sprouts, rinsed
   and drained

Cut the avocados in half and remove the stones (pits). Place the cut sides down and score the skin with the tip of a sharp knife down the middle. You should now be able to gently pull off the skins in two pieces, leaving the pear halves intact. Next, divide the sprouts evenly between four serving plates, flatten the mounds a little and gently loosen them. Place an avocado half on top of the sprouts and cut it across into slices, holding it together with the other hand. Push gently to fan out the slices evenly. Pour the sauce on top and sprinkle with the remaining seeds. Serve as a lunch or first course.

 As always, choosing the perfect avocado is the difference between heaven and dreadful disappointment. Choose them evenly green and giving to slight pressure at the stem end. The black knobbly type, or hass, is trickier to judge as the skins are very hard even when the fruit is soft inside. If they are hard in the shop, buy them anyway and wait 3–4 days before making this dish, while the avocado ripens to perfection in your kitchen.

CREAMED CÉLERI-RAVE

900g/2lb potatoes, peeled and chopped

900g/2lb celeriac (celery root), peeled and chopped

2 medium onions, chopped, with a couple of layers
   of golden skin reserved

½ teaspoon grated nutmeg

½ teaspoon ground black pepper

1 teaspoon low-salt bouillon powder

300ml (10 fl oz/1¼ cups) soya milk

water, to cover

Bring to the boil and simmer until the potatoes and celeriac (celery root) are very soft, 20–25 minutes. The onion skin will add a golden glow to the colour. Drain and discard the onion skin, then mash the vegetables to a smooth purée. You can do this in a blender or food processor or, best of all, through a *mouli passoir* – a gadget with a handle attached to a blade that pushes the goodies down through little holes to make the smoothest mash ever.

chopped fresh parsley or chives, to serve

Sprinkle with parsley or chives and serve hot.

 I like the sound of the French name *céleri boule* for celeriac (celery root), which I mix with potatoes and use instead of ordinary mash. If you like, you can stir the liquid back into the purée and heat through to make a delicious soup.

FUN, FIRE AND DELIGHT

4 medium yellow-fleshed sweet potatoes, pricked
    with a fork
4 medium onions, whole in their skins
4 whole bulbs fresh garlic, choose ones with
    big cloves

Wrap the vegetables individually in foil and nestle them in the hot ashes of a wood fire. If you don't mind brushing the bits off, the foil is not necessary. The timing should be about 50 minutes, but you will need to pay attention and possibly turn them so they cook evenly.

When everything is giving the soft squeeze, you can prepare as follows or just let everyone have the fun of doing their own ...

hot bread – optional

Split open the sweet potatoes.

Snip the tops off the onions and split the skins from top to bottom with scissors or a sharp knife. Slip the juicy, sweet and steaming flesh from the skins.

Snip the tops off the garlic bulbs, separate the cloves and squeeze the flesh out on to the potatoes or hot bread.

4 tablespoons (¼ cup) tamari soy sauce
2 tablespoons olive oil
pinch of ground black pepper
4 tablespoons (¼ cup) dry roasted sesame seeds,
    coarsely ground
juice of 1 lime – optional
some chopped fresh parsley

Combine and sprinkle on top of the pile of hot prepared vegetables, or pass separately for self-assembly.

 There is no doubt that even the most simple of foods are elevated to the realms of heavenly delight when cooked amongst the smoke and fragrance of a fire in the open air. If you do not happen to have a bonfire of smouldering wood and ashes to hand, try this in a 220°C/425°F/Gas 7 oven. Place everything just as it is on a baking (cookie) tray and bake for about 50 minutes.

GARLIC SOUP

6 tablespoons olive oil

40 cloves garlic from about 3 whole fresh bulbs,
   peeled

2 medium potatoes, peeled and chopped

1 small carrot, finely chopped

1.5 litres (2½ pints/1½ quarts) stock made
   with water and 1 tablespoon low-salt
   bouillon powder

Warm the oil in a large pan and add the garlic.
Cover and heat gently for a few minutes. Stir
in the potatoes and carrot and add the stock.
Simmer gently, uncovered, for about 25
minutes until the vegetables are very soft.
Cool a little, then whizz to a smooth cream in a
blender or food processor.

 Nice sprinkled with parsley and with hot brown bread.

Take heart and make this for your heart and soul. The texture is like velvet and the taste mellow
and sweet. The more garlic you use the smoother the cream, without much change in the flavour,
so be courageous. The fresher the garlic the sweeter the soup.

GENTLE ONION SAUCE

4 medium onions, roughly sliced

1 medium potato, peeled and diced

2 bay leaves

4 whole cloves

½ teaspoon ground black pepper

1 teaspoon low-salt yeast extract

2 teaspoons low-salt bouillon powder

sprig of rosemary

900ml (1½ pints/3¾ cups) soya milk

Just simmer gently together in a big heavy
pan, covered, for about 30 minutes until
onions are really soft. Remove the bits and
pieces and whizz in a blender or food
processor until smooth.

 You can use this sauce for a gratin or try it with Sage and Onion Sausages (see page 88).

INDONESIAN SPROUT
AND NUT SALAD

2 tablespoons light tahini	Combine to a smooth dressing in a large salad
1 tablespoon roasted sesame oil – optional	bowl.
1 green chilli, finely chopped – optional	
juice of 1 lemon	
2 teaspoons tamari soy sauce	
4 fresh mint leaves, finely chopped	
2 tablespoons peanut butter	
pinch of ground black pepper	
little splash of cider vinegar	

100g (4oz/¾ cup) plain peanuts or cashews	Fry in a dry pan over a moderate heat until they begin to turn golden. Or roast them on a baking (cookie) sheet in the oven. Add to the dressing while still warm.

½ cucumber, finely chopped or grated	Gently toss into the nuts and dressing and
3–4 handfuls of mung bean sprouts or chick pea (garbanzo bean) sprouts or your favourite mixture.	serve immediately. Sprinkle with fresh coriander (cilantro) if you can.
2–3 radishes, finely chopped or grated	
some chopped fresh coriander (cilantro), if you have it	

 This salad is delicious on its own, or when quickly stirred into hot brown rice. Raw vegetables and hot grains make a wonderful one-bowl lunch.

RED ONION RELISH

5 medium red onions, cut in half then finely sliced *5 tablespoons olive oil* *1 teaspoon ground black pepper* *4 juniper berries*	Soften together in heavy pan. Cover and cook without browning for 10 minutes.

200ml (7 fl oz/scant 1 cup) cider vinegar or red *wine vinegar* *4 tablespoons (¼ cup) runny honey* *2 tablespoons tamari soy sauce*	Add to the onions and simmer uncovered for 45 minutes. Keep the heat very low and stir occasionally. Cool to serve – it should have the consistency of a slightly runny jam.

 A handy little chutney that will liven up anything. It keeps very well in a jar in the fridge.

BASIL AND GARLIC ROASTED RED ROOTS

OVEN: 180°C/350°F/GAS 4

4 apple-size raw beetroots (beets), peeled and each one cut into 8 pieces
4 cloves garlic, halved lengthways
handful of fresh basil leaves
sprinkle of freshly ground black pepper
1 tablespoon olive oil

Put everything on a sheet of foil or into a roasting bag. Wrap, making sure all of the edges are sealed, then bake in the oven for 35–40 minutes.

Beetroots (beets) and basil are a match made in heaven – the aroma as you unwrap the package is truly divine. If you have some left over, slice it, splash with a little cider vinegar and pile it into a fresh brown bread sandwich. Delicious.

These incredibly coloured roots are not only scrumptious but also rich in iron, potassium, niacin, copper and vitamin C, with some extra folic acid, zinc, calcium, manganese, magnesium and phosphorus.

If you have been discouraged from eating beetroots (beets) by the vinegar-pickled kind, do try again as you will be pleasantly surprised by just how delicious they become when roasted in this way.

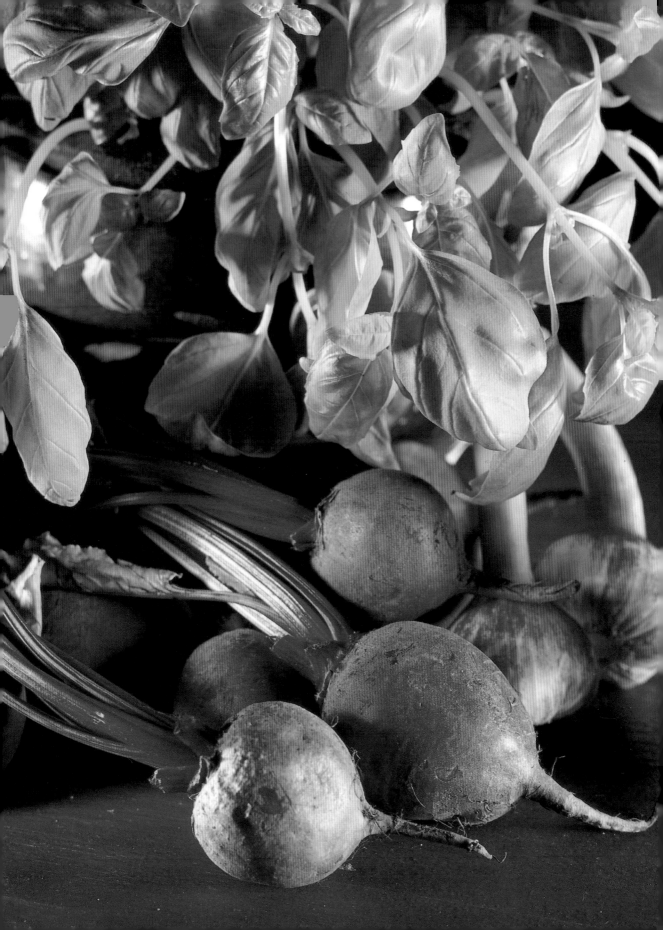

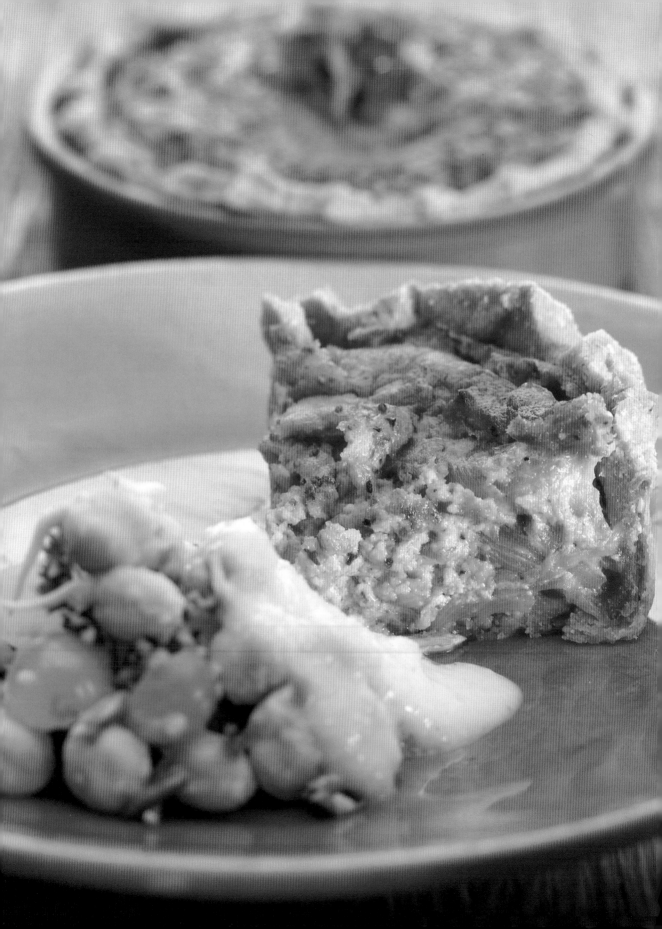

ONION TARTE

OVEN: 200°C/400°F/GAS 6

150g (5oz/1 cup) wholemeal (wholewheat) flour
100g (4oz/¾ cup) organic white flour
50g (2oz/¼ cup) soya margarine
3 tablespoons olive oil
1 teaspoon tamari soy sauce
1 teaspoon sesame seeds
cold water, to mix

Mix the flours in a bowl and rub in the fats. Add the tamari and sesame seeds and enough water to form a pliable pastry. Chill and use to line a 25cm/10 inch loose-bottomed quiche pan. Keep cold.

5 medium onions, sliced
4 tablespoons (¼ cup) olive oil
small sprig of rosemary
1 teaspoon ground nutmeg
½ teaspoon ground black pepper

Soften together in a frying pan for 10 minutes, then increase the heat to evaporate the juices and begin to caramelize the onions.

2 tablespoons tamari soy sauce
2 tablespoons soya milk
225g (8oz/1 cup) plain silken tofu
2 teaspoons Dijon mustard

Splash 2 teaspoons of the tamari over the hot onions. Beat or blend the rest into the milk, tofu and mustard. When smooth, quickly stir the mixture into the onions, tip into the pastry case and spread evenly. Bake in the oven for 10 minutes, then reduce the temperature to 180°C/350°F/Gas 4 and bake for a further 30 minutes. Keep an eye on it so that the top doesn't burn before the pastry is cooked.

A healthier variation of the French classic. Rich, sweet and more-ish.

If you like you can precook the pastry case, then just finish it with 15 minutes in a hot oven once the onion cream is in.

SPICY SPROUTED MUNG BEANS

4 tablespoons (¼ cup) olive oil
1 bay leaf
1 tablespoon whole black mustard seeds
¼ teaspoon asafetida powder – available from ethnic stores

Heat the oil with the bay leaf until the leaf is browning. Throw in the seeds and asafetida and let them pop for a couple of minutes (don't worry if it's a bit smoky).

1 medium onion, thinly sliced
1 teaspoon grated fresh root ginger
3 cloves garlic, grated

Stir into the pan, giving 3–4 minutes over a high heat. Reduce the heat, cover and cook for a further few minutes until the onion is soft and slushy.

1 teaspoon turmeric
½ teaspoon chilli powder – optional
½ teaspoon ground black pepper
juice of 1 big lemon
8 tablespoons (½ cup) water
350g (12oz/3 cups) mung bean sprouts, prepared as opposite

Stir the spices into the onions, cook for a minute or two and then add the remaining ingredients. Cover and cook gently for about 20 minutes. Check during cooking that all the liquid hasn't disappeared – you may need a little more.

handful of fresh coriander (cilantro) leaves
2 spring onions (scallions), shredded, or a little raw onion, chopped
2 teaspoons lemon juice – optional, to taste
1 fresh green chilli, finely chopped – optional
2 teaspoons tamari soy sauce – optional

Scatter on top just before serving.

Good with cooked grains or scooped with pitta bread or chapatis.

Bean sprouts are very popular in certain styles of Indian cookery – the sprouts are used at a much earlier stage of development than the more familiar Chinese ones that are left longer to become white and crisp. For this recipe, soak the mung beans overnight, rinse and leave in a jar (see page 18) in a dark place until the following day, rinsing twice. The beans will have sprouted little short tails and be ready to use. Pick out any that have not sprouted – they usually sink as you give them a final wash in a bowl of water.

STIR-FRY OF BABY LEEKS AND SPROUTS

---

2 tablespoons olive oil
3 star anise
3 cloves garlic, grated
5cm/2 inch piece of fresh root ginger, grated
1 dried red chilli, chopped or crumbled – optional

Sizzle together in a very hot wok.

750g (1½lb) young leeks, trimmed and cut into
  diagonal slices

Keep the heat up and add to the wok, shaking and stirring and making lots of noise and steam for 5 minutes. Lower the heat, cover and cook for 5 more minutes.

3–4 handfuls or as many as you want of sprouted
  chick peas (garbanzo beans)
1 tablespoon tamari soy sauce
pinch of ground black pepper

Add to the wok and increase the heat again, sizzle and mix thoroughly. Remove from the heat.

 Smooth leeks and crunchy sprouts – a lovely combination. Serve with noodles or rice.

BURIED TREASURES

Root foods buried in the earth have the advantage of being perfectly designed 'store cupboards' of nutrients. Of course they're not intended to be for our protection and delight, but to grow and sustain a glorious sun-feeding plant. Treasure them for their high content of vitamin A, vitamin C, iron, phosphorus, calcium, vitamin B, fibre and energy-providing carbohydrates.

These wonderful vegetables are invaluable in a healthy diet, not only for their nutrients but also for their wonderful array of flavours and textures. Each one has a different package of goodies to offer, so be adventurous and try new kinds when you see them. The good old potato is so versatile and of course so too is the carrot – ever changing from tiny, finger-size golden babies to the rich sweet giants of midwinter. Go ahead and experiment with sweet potatoes, beetroot (beets), radish, Jerusalem artichokes, yams, parsnips, swede (rutabaga) and turnips.

JERUSALEM ARTICHOKE AND WATERCRESS SOUP

2 tablespoons olive oil

1 medium onion, finely chopped

450g/1lb Jerusalem artichokes, scrubbed or peeled and sliced

Heat the oil in a large heavy pan and sauté gently until the onion is soft and transparent.

900ml (1½ pints/3¾ cups) vegetable stock or water

2 teaspoons low-salt bouillon powder

150ml (5 fl oz/⅔ cup) soya milk

good handful or bunch of fresh watercress

Whizz together in a blender or food processor or with a hand blender. Add about one-third of the vegetables from the pan and whizz again. Return to the pan and heat through. Do not boil.

grated zest (peel) of ½ lemon

1 teaspoon miso paste or low-salt yeast extract

½ teaspoon ground black pepper

Stir into the soup and serve.

 Sometimes try fresh parsley or basil instead of watercress.

WINTER VEGGIE TARTE TATIN

SERVES 6–8
OVEN: 190°C/375°F/GAS 5

300g (10oz/2 cups) large carrots, scrubbed or
   peeled and cut into thick round slices
300g (10oz/2 cups) parsnips, peeled and cut into
   round slices of the same thickness
3 tablespoons olive oil
1 bay leaf

Sauté together over a high heat in a heavy pan. When just browning, lower the heat and cover tightly. Cook very gently with a splash of water for 15 minutes. Uncover and set aside to cool.

100g (4oz/scant 1 cup) organic white flour
100g (4oz/scant 1 cup) wholemeal (wholewheat)
   flour
85g (3oz/6 tablespoons) soya margarine
3 tablespoons olive oil
cold water, to mix

Combine the flours in a bowl and rub in the fats until the mixture resembles breadcrumbs. Add water and knead to a flexible shortcrust pastry. Wrap and chill.

450g/1lb leeks, washed and shredded
25g (1oz/2 tablespoons) soya margarine

Soften together over a gentle heat and then cover, lower the heat and cook for 10 minutes. Do not brown. Tip into a blender or food processor with the following ingredients …

225g (8oz/1 cup) plain silken tofu
2 tablespoons tamari soy sauce
1 tablespoon soya milk
good grind of black pepper
good grating of nutmeg

… whizz until smooth.

Line a baking (cookie) tray measuring approximately 35 x 30cm/15 x 12 inches with a piece of non-stick baking parchment and carefully arrange the cooked root vegetables on it in an even flat layer that covers the whole tray. Pour the leek mixture on top, spread evenly and tap the tray two or three times to ensure that the creamy leeks fill any spaces. Roll out the pastry and lay over the whole tray. Make sure it goes right to the edge, but there is no need to press or seal around.

Bake in the oven for 35–40 minutes. Leave to stand for 5 minutes before carefully covering with another tray and inverting. Gently peel off the paper.

Serve with salad and/or green leafy vegetables.

This 'upside-down' method of producing a crisp tart is usually reserved for the luscious French apple version. It works very well here and once you have mastered the knack, I urge you to experiment with different root vegetables.

Don't be put off by the turning-over bit at the last minute. Just make sure that your serving tray is a bit bigger than your baking (cookie) tray, wear oven gloves (mitts), grasp the tray firmly at each end and turn it over in one confident movement.

You can halve the quantities and make it in a quiche pan or flan tin. Alternatively, make two and freeze one just before the final baking stage. Thaw to cook.

LOTTIE BAKE

OVEN: 180°C/350°F/GAS 4

8 tablespoons (½ cup) olive oil

large sprig of fresh thyme or 1 teaspoon
    dried thyme

twig of fresh rosemary

1 tablespoon tomato paste

2 medium onions, each one cut into about
    8 fat wedges

8 cloves garlic, whole or to your taste

2 medium carrots, each cut into 6 fingers

2 sweet potatoes or equivalent amount of squash,
    marrow (vegetable marrow) or courgette
    (zucchini)

8 small Jerusalem artichokes or peeled chopped
    celeriac (celery root) or both

2 medium potatoes, each cut into quarters, or 8
    whole new potatoes instead

1 lemon, quartered

½ teaspoon ground black pepper

Get the oil hot in a big ovenproof pan. Toss in the herbs for a quick sizzle and then stir in the tomato paste. Add all the other ingredients, stir and mix well. Cover and place in the oven for 40 minutes. Check once during this time, give it a good scrape off the bottom of the pan and stir gently. The vegetables should be soft after 40 minutes, so uncover and leave in the oven for another 15 minutes to get nice and 'roasty'. If you find that the veggies are not quite soft, splash with a little water and cook covered for a bit longer. Just before serving, squeeze the juices from the lemon pieces with the back of a spoon and stir gently. The lemon will be soft and delicious.

 Sprinkle with a little tamari if you like, and enjoy with salad.

For many happy years I was lucky enough to share a beautiful house with a dear friend. Not only did she cope with a huge house, a garden with ever-threatening ground elder and four boisterous children, she also struggled valiantly with an allotment (vegetable garden) – attempting to supply home-grown organic vegetables for her very abundant kitchen. The allotment was affectionately known as 'Lottie' and this dish became a favourite way of using almost anything that made its weary way home in the wheelbarrow. It is well worth a try with any combination of vegetables that you have to hand.

POTATOES WITH WHITE POPPY SEEDS

450g/1lb potatoes, peeled and cut into pieces about the size of a walnut	Cook in boiling water for about 15 minutes until just soft. Drain.
8 teaspoons white poppy seeds *1 tablespoon water*	Grind to a rough paste in a pestle and mortar.
1 medium onion, finely chopped *6 tablespoons light olive oil* *1 teaspoon turmeric* *pinch of chilli powder – optional* *approximately 4 tablespoons (¼ cup) water*	Soften the onion in the oil over a gentle heat. When the onion is really soft and slushy, add the spices and continue to cook, stirring very gently, for 4–5 minutes. Mix in the poppy-seed paste, add the water and cooked potatoes and stir thoroughly. Cover and cook very gently until the potatoes are really soft. You may need to add a little more water to stop them sticking.
1 tablespoon tamari soy sauce *1 green chilli, finely chopped – optional* *1 tablespoon mustard oil – available in Asian stores, but optional*	Sprinkle on top.

Serve with Spinach Chapatis (see page 70) and a tomato and onion salad.

In India this delicious little bit of magic with potatoes is known as *alu posto*. I have persuaded my father to give me this recipe as his version is by far the best I have ever eaten.

White poppy seeds are small and ivory-coloured, usually available in Asian stores. High in calcium like their bigger 'blue' brothers, they have a subtle and unique flavour and a strangely satisfying texture. The blue-black seeds are more readily available but they do not work well in this dish, so wait until you come across the white ones, sometimes sold under the name of *khus khus*.

ONION AND POTATO PAKORAS

OVEN: 190°C/375°F/GAS 5

3 medium onions, very finely sliced

1 medium potato, coarsely grated

few sprigs of fresh coriander (cilantro) leaves, chopped

½ teaspoon black onion seeds or nigella seeds

1 tablespoon olive oil

1 tablespoon tamari soy sauce – optional

Combine in a large bowl.

100g (4oz/scant 1 cup) gram flour (besan, chick pea flour, channa flour)

Sift into the bowl and knead with your hand for about 5 minutes until well mixed. The juices will come out of the onions and be absorbed by the flour to form a 'glue'. All the pieces of onion and potato should have some of the batter sticking to them, so if your onions are very juicy you may need to sprinkle in more flour. You can't put too much flour in as long as you don't have any dry powdery bits. The mix should be quite stiff.

olive oil, for frying

Heat some oil in a shallow frying pan (a non-stick pan will mean you can use less oil). Place spoonfuls of the mix carefully into the oil, flatten the tops down a bit and fry over a moderate heat for about 5 minutes on each side. Do a few at a time and keep them on a baking (cooking) tray in the oven until you have cooked them all. The size is up to you, but don't make them too thick or the potato will not be cooked in the middle.

 A little crispy snack with salad, salsa and/or rice and dhal.

DAIRY FREE DAUPHINOIS

OVEN: 189°C/350°F/GAS 4

450g/1lb carrots, thinly sliced

1.4 kg/3lb large floury potatoes, peeled if you like and sliced thicker

Bring to the boil in a large pan of boiling water and cook for 8 minutes. Drain and tip into a greased large ovenproof dish. Shake and settle the vegetables down – the dish should be about half full.

If you put a couple of bay leaves or a sprig of thyme or rosemary in the bottom of the dish, so much the better.

175g (6oz/heaping 1 cup) plain cashew nut pieces

1 litre (1¾ pints/1 quart) soya milk

4 cloves garlic, more if you like

1 teaspoon grated nutmeg

4 teaspoons low-salt bouillon powder

1 teaspoon ground black pepper

Whizz until smooth in a blender or food processor. Depending on the power of your machine, it is sometimes worth giving the nuts a quick whizz on their own first to avoid lumps. Pour the resulting cream over the vegetables in the dish and give it a wriggle to mix thoroughly. Cover and bake in the oven for 40 minutes.

a little olive oil or soya margarine

Uncover and drizzle with a little olive oil or dot with soya margarine. Bake uncovered for a further 15 minutes until soft and well browned.

When I stopped eating dairy food I really missed the French classic *gratin dauphinois.* I am almost embarrassed to say that in my early years of training with French chefs we used to make one for an evening in the restaurant using 6 litres (10 pints/6 quarts) double (heavy) cream. This version gives the same satisfying richness, but with less strain on the heart. I have added carrots for flavour and prettiness, but it works well with just potatoes or other mixtures of root vegetables.

THAI GREEN CURRY OF SWEET POTATOES AND QUORN

2 green chillies, deseeded and chopped

2.5cm/1 inch piece of fresh root ginger, grated

1 teaspoon ground black pepper

1 small onion, chopped

5 cloves garlic, chopped

50g (2oz/1 cup) fresh coriander (cilantro), chopped

grated zest (peel) of 1 big lemon

2 teaspoons ground coriander

1 teaspoon ground cumin

1 teaspoon turmeric

1 tablespoon olive oil

2 tablespoons water

Place in a blender or food processor and purée. You will probably have to stop to scrape down the sides a few times. If it is reluctant, add a tiny bit more oil.

---

3 tablespoons oil

2 small onions, each cut into about 6 thick wedges

3 medium sweet potatoes, peeled and each cut into about 8 pieces

Heat the oil in a pan, toss in the onions and stir well, then add the sweet potatoes. Stir well, keep it sizzling and mix in the green curry paste. Cook gently for 5 minutes, stirring occasionally.

600ml (1 pint/2½ cups) coconut milk

a few kaffir lime leaves – optional

12cm/5 inch stem of lemon grass – optional

2 tablespoons tamari soy sauce

Add to the pan. The liquid should cover the vegetables by about 2.5cm/1 inch, so you may need to top up with water. Simmer slowly for 20 minutes.

225g (8oz/2 cups) plain quorn pieces

juice of ½ lemon

Add to the pan and continue simmering very slowly, partially covered, for a further 15 minutes. The potatoes should be soft and the sauce rich.

Lovely served over plain brown rice and broccoli.

I don't often use quorn, as to some extent it is a processed food. Having said that, there are some dishes like this one that it works very well for – and it is an excellent source of protein, but only occasionally. It does make a change in this dish but it will work happily without it.

This curry is pretty hot, so if your tastebuds can be a bit delicate, reduce the chilli.

BRAISED ROOTS

2 tablespoons olive oil

3 carrots, scrubbed or peeled and cut into 2.5cm/
   1 inch pieces

1 small swede (rutabaga), peeled and cut into
   chunks

about the same amount of turnips, cut into
   similar-size pieces

2 medium parsnips, peeled and cut into
   similar-size pieces

½ teaspoon ground black pepper

sprig of fresh thyme

Heat the oil in a large heavy pan and toss in everything else. Stir well over a high heat until the vegetables are almost beginning to brown. Reduce the heat to very, very low, splash in 2 tablespoons water and cover tightly. Cook for 20 minutes, shaking or stirring occasionally until the carrots are soft.

 This method of cooking really does transform and intensify the sweetness and flavour of the most humble of vegetables.

WARMING SWEET POTATO CASSEROLE

OVEN: 180°C/350°F/GAS 4

6 tablespoons olive oil

2 bay leaves

1 tablespoon dried basil

5cm/2 inch piece of fresh root ginger, grated

½ teaspoon chilli powder – optional, to taste

1 teaspoon whole coriander seeds, crushed

1 medium onion, grated

1 medium carrot, grated

1 sweet red pepper (bell pepper), very finely
chopped

Heat the oil and herbs together in a heavy pan, add the remaining ingredients and stir well. Lower the heat, cover and soften gently for 10 minutes. Watch out for burning.

2 teaspoons tomato paste

1 tablespoon tamari soy sauce

6 large tomatoes, finely chopped, or 1 x 400g/
14oz can

approximately 300ml (10 fl oz/1¼ cups) creamy
coconut milk or

50g (2oz/¼ cup) chopped creamed coconut,
dissolved in 300ml (10 fl oz/1¼ cups) boiling
water

Stir the tomato paste and tamari into the vegetables and cook and stir for 3–4 minutes before adding the tomatoes. Cook and stir again over a gentle heat for 5 minutes, then add the coconut and stir well.

approximately 900g/2lb red-skinned, yellow-
fleshed sweet potatoes, peeled and sliced into
thick rounds

Layer in an oiled casserole dish. It should be about half full.

Pour the sauce over the top and wriggle the dish to spread it evenly to the bottom.

2 tablespoons tamari soy sauce	Splash and sprinkle over the casserole and
1 tablespoon olive oil	bake in the oven for approximately 40 minutes
1 teaspoon ground black pepper	until the potatoes are really soft and the top is
	bubbly and golden. You can speed this up if
	you parboil the potato slices for 10 minutes at
	the beginning.

 This method also works well using ordinary potatoes and celeriac (celery root) or squash, or a mixture of roots.

Serve with chunks of wholemeal (wholewheat) bread and a green vegetable or salad.

MY MUM'S PERFECT CARROTS

3 tablespoons olive oil	Heat the oil and throw in the carrots. Toss
4 large carrots, scrubbed or peeled and thinly sliced	around over a high heat and keep stirring until they just begin to brown.

2 cloves garlic, finely chopped	Add to the pan and sizzle madly for a minute
1 tablespoon water	or two. Reduce the heat, cover tightly and
1 tablespoon cider or wine vinegar	cook gently for 15–20 minutes. The carrots
2 teaspoons tamari soy sauce – optional	will be soft and the liquid mostly absorbed.
pinch of ground black pepper	

handful of fresh parsley or basil, chopped	Gently stir into the carrots and serve hot or cold.

 So simple, yet never quite as good as hers.

GRATIN OF ROOTS WITH A TWIST

OVEN: 200°C/400°F/GAS 6

4 medium potatoes, scrubbed or peeled and cut
  into quarters
450g/1lb swede (rutabaga), peeled and chopped
225g (8oz/heaping 1½ cups) carrots, cut into quite
  thin rounds
a little sprig of fresh thyme or 1 teaspoon
  dried thyme
8 juniper berries, crushed or bruised with the back
  of a spoon
2 bay leaves
4 teaspoons low-salt bouillon powder
300ml (10 fl oz/1¼ cups) water
600ml (1 pint/2½ cups) soya milk

Put everything into a large pan and simmer until the potatoes are just soft (approximately 20 minutes after coming to the boil). The liquid should cover the vegetables by about 2.5cm/1 inch – this will depend on the shape of your pan and you may need to top it up with water or soya milk.

juice of 1 lemon
25g (1oz/2 tablespoons) soya margarine

Put a colander over a large bowl and strain the roots, reserving all the liquid. Tip one-third of the vegetables back into the pan with the liquid and boil uncovered for a further 10 minutes.

Put the rest of the vegetables into an ovenproof dish. Pour the lemon juice over them and dot with the margarine.

Blend or mash the roots and liquid left in the pan to create a smooth sauce. If you use an electric blender or food processor, remove the twigs, berries and leaves first. Pour the sauce over the vegetables to just about cover (if you have some left over, freeze it or use it for soup or stock).

Bake the gratin in the oven for 20 minutes or brown carefully under the grill (broiler).

 Try serving this with Green Beans with Garlic and Almonds (see page 139).

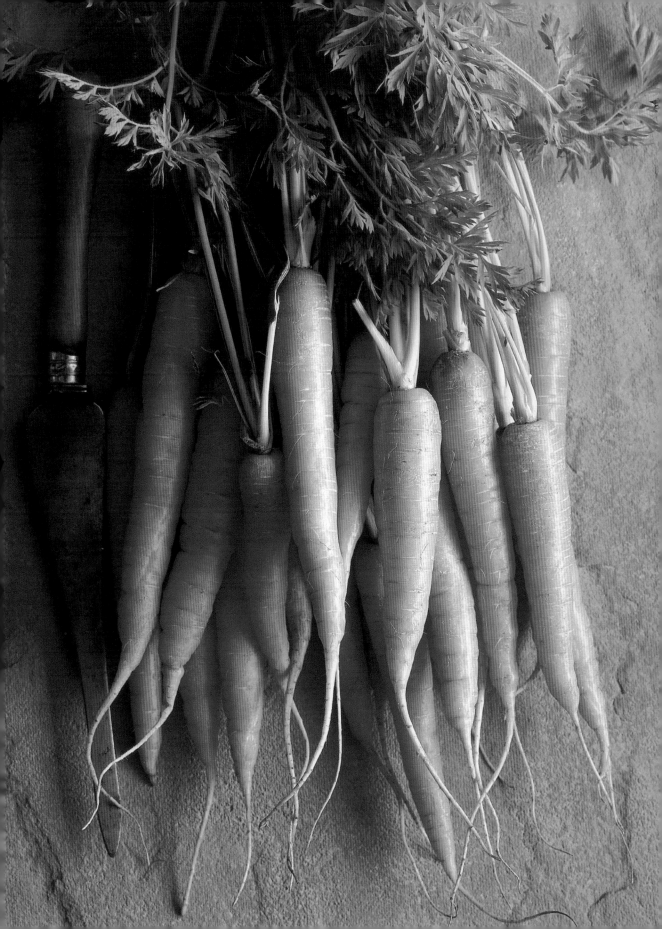

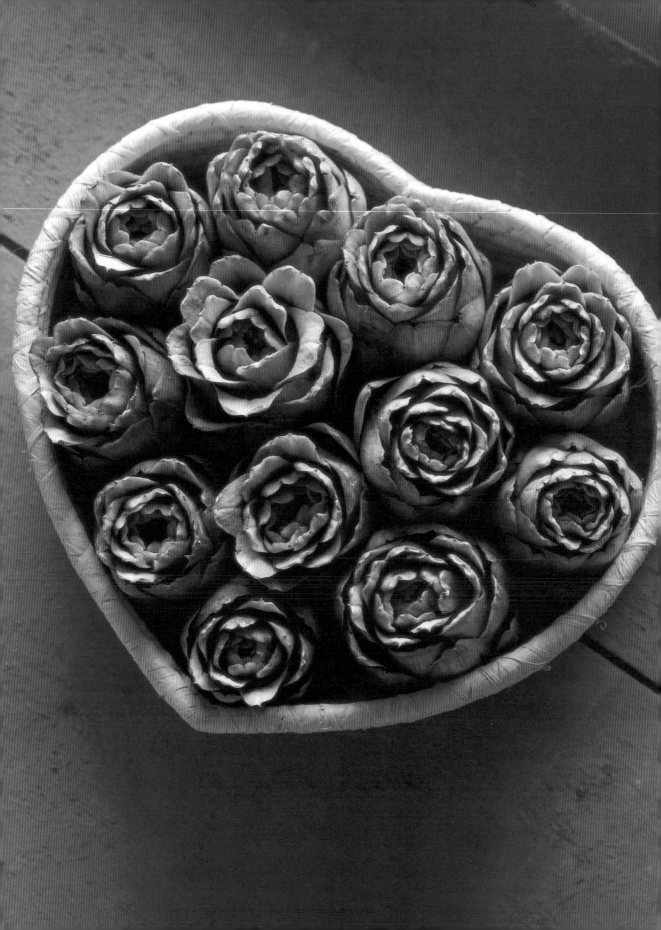

DARLING BUDS

Somehow, just the very notion of eating the buds of flowers sends my mind off into thoughts of billowing clouds, shafts of sunlight and the ethereal world of the Greek gods and goddesses. Tender, tiny and holding the promise of millions of soft petals – surely a divine, luxuriant food for angels.

My reasons for including them here are, of course, not entirely whimsical. Many flower buds are good sources of nutrients, vitamin C and folic acid, and are plentiful providers of potassium. Broccoli is especially rich in betacarotene, vitamin C, calcium and a good range of minerals with some iron. Both broccoli and cauliflower are good sources of protein and are members of the cruciferous family, well known for its cancer-preventing qualities.

Globe artichokes and asparagus are renowned for having great beneficial effects on our kidneys, liver and digestive system. They are wonderful purifying and detoxifying foods.

So, flower buds to include regularly in your meals are broccoli (calabrese), purple and white sprouting broccoli, cauliflower and cape cauliflower (these are the perfectly formed spirals of lime green or dark purple), globe artichokes and asparagus.

They are all perfect simply steamed until just soft, and they come into their own as the contrast to richer, fuller dishes.

Read on for other ideas with flower buds.

ARTICHOKES WITH MUSTARD SEED VINAIGRETTE

4 globe artichokes – see below for how to prepare
juice of ½ lemon

Drop the artichokes into a large pan of boiling water and weight them down with a plate if they float about. Cover and boil gently for 35–40 minutes. A middle leaf will pull out quite easily when they are cooked. Drain and serve warm or cold with or without the sauce.

300ml (10 fl oz/1¼ cups) olive oil
2 tablespoons yellow mustard seeds, soaked in
  cider vinegar overnight
3 tablespoons cider vinegar
1 tablespoon tamari soy sauce – or to your taste
½ teaspoon ground black pepper
splash of apple juice

Whizz in a blender or food processor and divide between four individual dishes so each person may dip his or her own artichoke into the sauce. Provide plates for the debris.

 Use artichokes of any size from a cricket ball to a melon. The bigger they are, the longer they take to cook. To prepare them, trim off the top third and the pointy bits with scissors, then level the stem to the base so it can sit up straight on the plate.

Eating artichokes in this way can be a delightful meditation for a quiet lunch alone or fun with friends and children. Pull the leaves off one by one and use your teeth to pull off the sweet flesh. The leaves get softer as you make your way in, until you can pull out the cluster in the middle and nibble round the edge. Pull out the hairy choke – don't eat any hairs however enthusiastic you may be to get at the succulent base beneath.

I always keep a small jar of vinegar-soaked mustard seeds in the fridge as they are a great addition to dressings and keep for ages.

ASPARAGUS WITH MARINATED ONIONS

12 fat spring onions (scallions), trimmed and cut in half lengthways

4 tablespoons (¼ cup) olive oil

2 teaspoons Dijon mustard

1 teaspoon balsamic vinegar or lemon or lime juice

2 teaspoons fresh thyme leaves, finely chopped

1 teaspoon tamari soy sauce

good pinch of ground black pepper

Combine carefully and leave to marinate for about 1 hour.

16 asparagus spears (4 per person), washed and any tough ends removed

Drop into boiling water and cook 5 minutes until a sharp knife point will easily slip through the fat ends. Drain and allow them to sit in the onion marinade for a few minutes, so they are well covered with the juices. Lift the vegetables from the marinade and lay them in a flameproof shallow dish or grill (broiler) pan. Cook under a very hot grill (broiler) for 5 minutes on each side, or in a hot dry pan or griddle for 3–4 minutes on each side.

Cut into smaller pieces to serve warm on a cushion of mixed leaves, or just lay them on individual serving plates and serve as they are. Drizzle with any remaining marinade to serve.

 If you are lucky enough to find little baby leeks you can use them instead of onions.

BROCCOLI PASTA ARRABBIATA

450g/1lb broccoli, cut into florets and tender stems, chopped

Drop into boiling water and cook for 5 minutes until the stems are just soft. Drain.

225g (8oz/2⅔ cups) dried pasta shells or spirals or spaghetti – I like to use half wholemeal (wholewheat) and half green

Cook according to package instructions. Drain.

5 tablespoons olive oil
2 teaspoons dried or fresh red chillies, or more or less according to your taste, finely chopped
4 cloves garlic, finely chopped
1 teaspoon ground black pepper
finely grated zest (peel) of 1 lemon or lime

Heat the oil in a large pan and throw in everything else. Sizzle and stir until the garlic just begins to brown – this should hardly take a minute.

Add the broccoli and pasta and keep stirring and shaking the pan to mix well and heat everything through.

3 ripe sweet tomatoes, finely chopped
handful of fresh parsley or basil leaves, roughly chopped
1 tablespoon tamari soy sauce – optional

Quickly stir through the pasta and serve piping hot.

 Arrabbiata means 'raging' in Italian – raging with red hot chilli peppers. Calm it to your own taste or leave out the chillies and use finely chopped sweet red pepper (bell pepper), or half of each, or even forget the whole hot thing and use sesame seeds instead.

STIR-FRIED ASPARAGUS WITH DATES AND CARROTS

2 tablespoons olive oil *1 teaspoon sesame oil* *5 star anise* *2.5cm/1 inch piece of fresh root ginger, grated*	Heat together in a wok over a high flame.
2 small onions, sliced *3 medium carrots, scrubbed or peeled and cut into very thin julienne (matchsticks)*	Add to the wok and keep the heat high while you shake and stir for a few minutes.
10–12 asparagus spears, trimmed and sliced – see below *8 fresh dates, cut into long strips* *½ teaspoon ground black pepper*	Add to the wok and keep the heat high while you shake and stir for a few minutes. Splash in a couple of spoonfuls of water and lower the heat. Cover and cook for 5 minutes.
3 tablespoons hot water *1 tablespoon miso paste* *1 teaspoon tamari soy sauce*	Combine in a cup until smooth, then add to the wok over a high heat. Stir and bubble, reduce the heat and cook for a couple more minutes before serving.

 The texture works well if the asparagus stems are sliced thinly and the tips are cut 5cm/2 inches long.

You can use dried dates – just give them a little soak beforehand.

Good with plain rice or noodles. Serve toasted and ground sesame seeds separately, for sprinkling over the dish at the table.

CAULIFLOWER BRAISED
IN SPICY CREAM

50g (2oz/⅔ cup) freshly grated coconut – see below

Toast until golden in a dry heavy frying pan. Tip into a blender or food processor.

85g (3oz/¾ cup) sesame seeds

Toast until golden in a dry heavy frying pan. Add to the coconut.

1 tablespoon olive oil
50g (2oz/scant ½ cup) plain cashew nut pieces
1 teaspoon whole cumin seeds
1 fresh green chilli, chopped, or to your taste
900ml (1½ pints/3¾ cups) water

Heat the oil and fry the nuts and seeds until browning. Add to the coconut and sesame seeds with the fresh chilli and water and whizz until fairly smooth.

2 tablespoons olive oil
1 tablespoon whole black mustard seeds
1 bay leaf
1 big cauliflower, cut into small bite-size pieces
*   including the tender leaves and stems*

Get the oil really hot and throw in the seeds and bay leaf. Let the seeds pop for a couple of seconds before adding the cauliflower. Stir well, spreading the seeds through the cauliflower for 4–5 minutes.

juice of 1 lemon
½ teaspoon ground black pepper
3 tablespoons tamari soy sauce – optional

Reduce the heat and add to the cauliflower with the sauce from the blender. Cover and cook gently for 15–20 minutes until the cauliflower is only just soft. Watch that it doesn't stick and stir and add a little more water if it begins to do so.

Sprinkle with a little more toasted coconut to serve. Try it with Basmati Green Terrine (see page 83) and a green salad tossed with a lemony dressing and grapes.

Fresh coconut is a must for this recipe. If you have never used one before, just wrap it in a cloth or a couple of layers of kitchen paper and give it a good sharp tap with a hammer or crack it open on a stone slab outside. It will break open into two or three pieces. Use a blunt knife to prise the white nut from the shell. It grates very easily. Some coconuts have a clear liquid inside – if you can save it, use it to replace some of the water in the recipe. Any leftover coconut can be sliced or grated, toasted and sprinkled over muesli or salads.

GREEN CAPER RELISH

50g (2oz/¼ cup) plain silken tofu
1 small lemon, deseeded and chopped
50g (2oz/1 cup) fresh parsley, roughly chopped
2 teaspoons cider vinegar
1 teaspoon tamari soy sauce – optional
pinch of ground black pepper
¼ medium cucumber, roughly chopped

Whizz in a blender or food processor.

---

3 tablespoons capers, finely chopped

Stir into the sauce.

Serve with any grilled (broiled) vegetables, or as a dressing for salads or warm new potatoes.

Capers are the tiny unopened flower buds of a little straggly spiny bush that can be found growing from the Mediterranean to the Gobi desert. The buds are usually pickled, and they add a nice zing to sauces and dressings.

MINTED CAULIFLOWER PURÉE

1 medium cauliflower, cut into florets, tender
leaves and stems chopped too
350g (12oz/2½ cups) shelled (podded) peas or
broad (fava) beans
few sprigs of fresh mint or 2 teaspoons dried mint
½ teaspoon grated nutmeg
pinch of ground black pepper
mixture of water and soya milk, to cover
1 teaspoon low-salt bouillon powder – optional

Bring to the boil and simmer about 20 minutes until the cauliflower is soft. Drain and whizz to a purée in a blender or food processor.

Garnish with extra fresh mint and a couple of dots of soya margarine to serve.

This is lovely with either peas or broad (fava) beans in the mix, but if you want a spectacularly bright green version, use the peas.

CAULIFLOWER CHEESE WITHOUT THE CHEESE

OVEN: 200°C/400°F/GAS 6

1 medium onion, finely chopped *1 bay leaf* *2 tablespoons olive oil* *1 tablespoon soya margarine*	Sauté gently together in a heavy pan until the onion is soft but not brown. Remove from the heat.
3 heaped tablespoons organic flour, white or brown, or a mixture of both	Stir into the pan to form a thick paste (a roux), then keep stirring until the mixture begins to come away from the sides of the pan.
900ml (1½ pints/3¾ cups) soya milk	Add slowly, stirring continuously, and return to a gentle heat. Keep stirring while it comes to the boil and thickens.
½ teaspoon grated nutmeg *1 tablespoon low-salt bouillon powder* *4 tablespoons nutritional yeast flakes* *½ teaspoon ground black pepper*	Stir into the sauce, mix well and cook for 5 minutes over a gentle heat. Cool slightly, then remove the bay leaf and whizz in a blender or food processor until smooth.
1 large cauliflower, cleaned and cut into florets, *olive oil and any seeds you have, for sprinkling*	Boil the cauliflower for 15 minutes in plenty of water. Drain and place in an ovenproof dish. Cover with the sauce, then splash with a little olive oil and a sprinkle of seeds. Bake in the oven for 20–25 minutes until well browned.

I am forever indebted to Adam Hynes, chef at the Bristol Cancer Help Centre, for persevering and experimenting until this sauce was perfect. He still makes the best ever.

I use it here as part of the well-loved old standby, but it is such a good basic sauce in a vegan kitchen and it seems to be endlessly versatile.

ORANGE BLASTED BROCCOLI

3 tablespoons olive oil finely grated zest (peel) of 2 big oranges 1 teaspoon fennel seeds – optional 50g (2oz/scant ½ cup) almonds – optional	Get the oil very hot in a wok and throw in the orange zest (peel) and fennel seeds. Sizzle for 2 seconds. Add the nuts.
750g/1½lb broccoli, cut into small pieces including tender stems and leaves ½ teaspoon ground black pepper	Add to the wok and stir-fry for 5 minutes.
juice of 2 big oranges 1 tablespoon tamari soy sauce	Pour over the broccoli and reduce the heat, then cover and cook for about 8 minutes until the broccoli is soft but with a little bite.

Garnish with fresh orange wedges, slices or segments and serve instantly.

FOREST FLOOR
AND SEABED

If you are someone who has only ever tried the type of white button mushrooms you get from the supermarket, and who is seriously unconvinced by the idea of eating seaweed, then I hope this chapter will give you the confidence to experiment and enjoy a wider range of these valuable foods.

Of course the button mushrooms we are all accustomed to are delicious in many dishes and can nearly always be used when others are not available. However, all types have a great deal of flavour and texture to offer and vary considerably in their nutrient content. Mushrooms contain protein, many of the B group of vitamins, potassium, sulphur and folic acid, while some are also quite high in iron and selenium.

Even with our well-loved, cultivated varieties the flavours and textures differ greatly with maturity and openness, but some others to look out for that have an especially good flavour are oyster mushrooms, chanterelles, shaggy parasol mushrooms, chestnut mushrooms and fresh or dried shiitake and ceps (porcini).

The chances are that even if you think you won't like sea vegetables (to describe them as weeds somehow seems to diminish their wonder), you will probably have eaten a pretty good quantity in your life without even realizing it. They contain carbohydrates known as phycocolloids that are extracted and used in many familiar packaged foods, including ice creams, jellies, soups, confectionery and sauces. Used as a vegetable, garnish or seasoning in their whole form, either fresh or dried, they can contribute immensely to flavour, and they can supply us with nutrients that are difficult to gain elsewhere. Japanese cooks have a range of about 50 species, but the ones we are most likely to encounter are arame, hijiki, dulse, kelp, kombu, nori and wakame. They are all rich in iodine, calcium, potassium and iron, with some high in protein as well. We would all be wise to start including ocean vegetables in our diet more regularly as they contain a fibre molecule (algin) which can bind with toxic metals from environmental pollutants and help eliminate these toxins from our bodies. Read the labels and always look for good-quality products from clean oceans.

RICH MUSHROOMS AND MASH

OVEN: 190°C/375°F/GAS 5

8 medium potatoes, peeled and diced 4 whole cloves garlic water, to cover	Boil until very soft. Drain.
150ml (5 fl oz/⅔ cup) soya milk ½ teaspoon ground nutmeg 6 spring onions (scallions), finely shredded	Mash milk and nutmeg into the potatoes until smooth and creamy, then stir in the onions (scallions). Keep warm.
1 medium onion, finely chopped 4 cloves garlic, sliced 1 bay leaf sprig or pinch of thyme 4 tablespoons (¼ cup) olive oil	Soften together in a heavy pan until the onion is transparent.
1 tablespoon tomato paste 450g/1lb button mushrooms, cleaned 25g (1oz/1 cup) dried porcini (ceps), soaked in 200ml (7 fl oz/scant 1 cup) hot water ½ teaspoon ground black pepper	Stir the tomato paste into the onion and let it sizzle for a minute before adding the mushrooms and juice and the pepper. Continue to cook and stir for 5 minutes over a high heat.
200ml (7 fl oz/scant 1 cup) organic red wine or red grape juice or a mixture – if you don't have the dried mushroom juice you may need a splash more 4 teaspoons tamari soy sauce juice of 1 orange 2 tablespoons malt extract (malt syrup) 4 teaspoons low-salt yeast	Add to the pan, bring to the boil and cook very gently for 15 minutes.

olive oil, for drizzling

In a separate bowl, carefully blend 1 cup of the sauce from the mushrooms with 1 cup of the mashed potato. Return the smooth mix to the mushrooms, mix and turn into an ovenproof dish. Depending on the shape of your dish, you may find you have a little too much gravy – just keep it warm in a jug to serve separately. Cover the mushrooms with the remaining mash and gently seal the edges. Drizzle with olive oil and brown in the oven for 15 minutes.

RAGOÛT OF WILD MUSHROOMS

4 tablespoons (¼ cup) olive oil

1 tablespoon soya margarine

½ teaspoon dried thyme or 1 sprig fresh thyme

½ teaspoon dried rosemary or 1 sprig fresh
  rosemary

450g/1lb any mixed mushrooms, cleaned and sliced
  – if you can include chanterelles or parasols in
  your mix the flavours are gorgeous

2 cloves garlic, crushed

½ teaspoon ground black pepper

Heat the oil, margarine and herbs in a large frying pan or wok until just smoking and then throw in everything else. Stir, sizzle and shake about for 5 minutes.

300ml (10 fl oz/1¼ cups) boiling water,
  including the soaking liquid if you have
  used a few dried mushrooms

2 teaspoons low-salt yeast extract

1 teaspoon low-salt bouillon powder

2 teaspoons malt extract (malt syrup)

Dissolve together and add to the pan. Allow to simmer and reduce a little for 6 minutes.

150g (5oz/1 cup) plain cashew nuts

300ml (10 fl oz/1¼ cups) soya milk

Whizz to a smooth cream in a blender or food processor, then add to the mushrooms. Stir well and simmer for 4–5 minutes until thick and creamy.

 Sprinkle with a little paprika if you have some and serve hot as a sauce over grains or pasta, or over a baked potato with broccoli.

If you find this dish just a little too creamy for your taste, squeeze in the juice of half a lemon just before serving for a more 'sour cream in the stroganoff' effect.

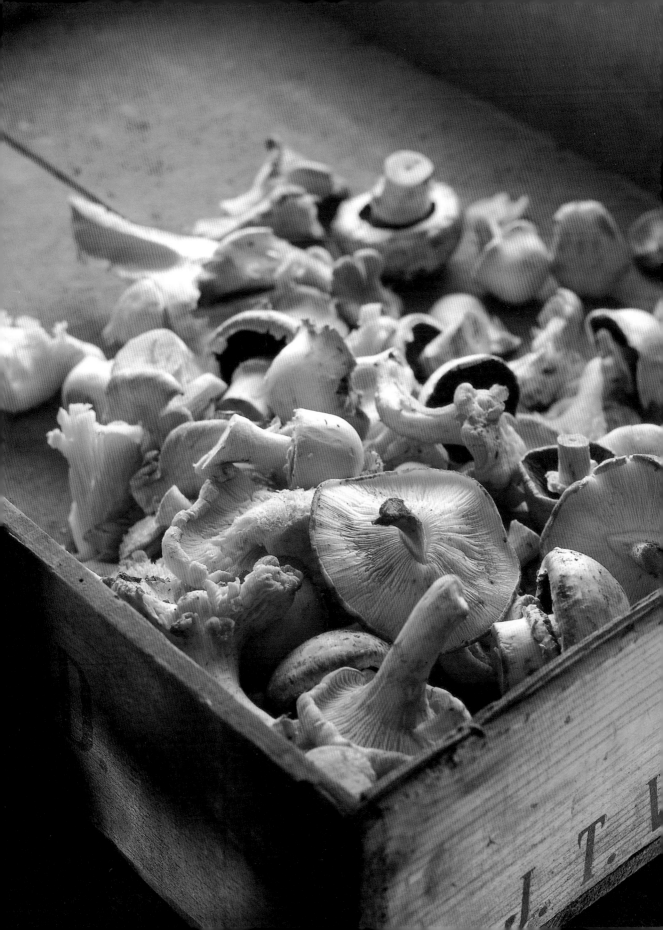

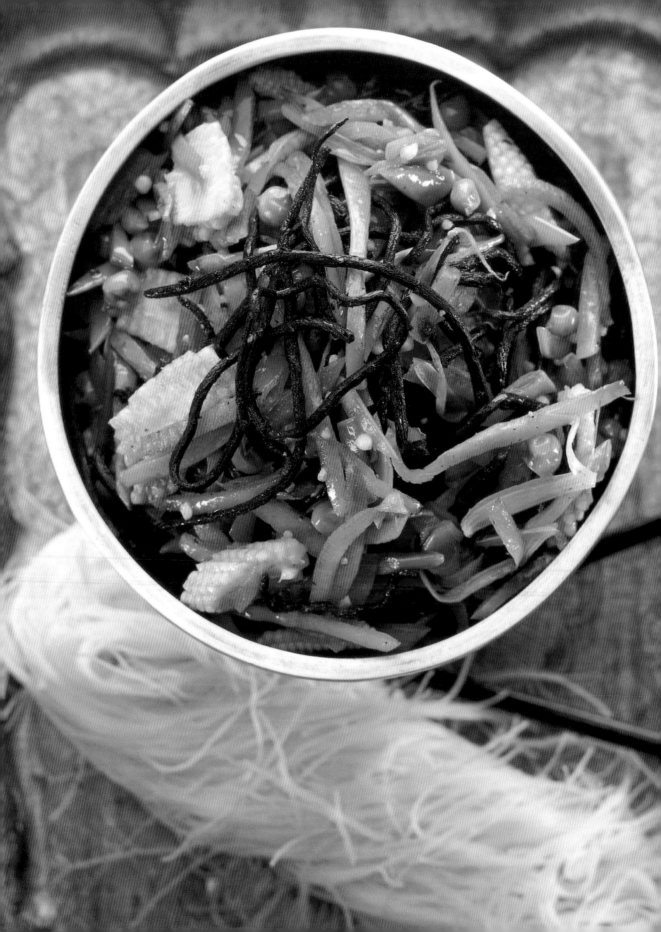

JAPANESE-STYLE HOT SALAD

25g (1oz/heaping ½ cup) dried hijiki seaweed,
   soaked in cold water for 30 minutes
2 teaspoons tamari soy sauce

Bring to the boil in the soaking water and boil for 5 minutes. Drain.

1 tablespoon olive oil
1 teaspoon roasted sesame oil
2 medium carrots, cut into very fine julienne
   (matchsticks)
2 spring onions (scallions), cut into fine strips

Heat the oils in a wok, add the vegetables and toss them around for a minute or two.

225g (8oz/2 cups) mangetout (snow peas), very
   finely shredded on the diagonal
100g (4oz/scant 1 cup) fresh or frozen peas
100g (4oz/heaping 1 cup) baby corn cobs, finely
   sliced on the diagonal

Keep the heat quite high and add the vegetables to the wok, stirring and shaking well to mix. Add the hijiki last.

1 tablespoon water
1 teaspoon cider vinegar or rice vinegar
1 tablespoon tamari soy sauce – optional
pinch of ground black pepper

Splash into the wok, sizzle for a second or two and serve.

 The whole process is pretty quick to cook in the wok as this is really a dish of hot raw vegetables rather than cooked. Try it with plain rice, buckwheat or rice noodles, or just as it is with chopsticks. It has very light and delicate flavours.

BROCCOLI AND POTATOES WITH SESAME AND ARAME

24 whole new potatoes *or 6 medium main-crop potatoes, each cut into* *quarters*	Leave the skins on and cook in plenty of boiling water until soft. Drain.
450g/1lb broccoli	Cut into bite-size florets and slice the tender stems. Plunge into boiling water for 5 minutes, drain and rinse in cold water.
2 tablespoons sesame seeds, roasted in a dry pan *for 5 minutes until popping and nutty* *3 tablespoons olive oil* *grated zest (peel) and juice of 1 lemon* *1 teaspoon grated fresh root ginger* *1 tablespoon tamari soy sauce* *1 teaspoon ground black pepper* *1 teaspoon light tahini – optional*	Combine in a large bowl.
25g (1oz/heaping ½ cup) dried arame sea *vegetable, soaked in cold water for 30 minutes*	Drain and stir into the dressing with the potatoes and broccoli. Serve warm or cool.

 I like this dish with the fine dark strands of arame, but it is just as delicious with the slightly thicker hijiki.

HERB-GRILLED GIANT PUFFBALL 'STEAKS'

1 football-size giant puffball mushroom

Wipe clean of any bits of field and cut off any little 'rooty' bit at the bottom. The skin is perfectly edible, but it allows for a very satisfying few minutes if you peel it. Cut into slices about as thick as your finger and lay them on a tray.

8 tablespoons (½ cup) olive oil
2 cloves garlic, crushed
2 tablespoons tamari soy sauce
1 teaspoon dried basil
½ teaspoon thyme leaves
pinch of ground black pepper

Combine in a small bowl and brush liberally on the puffball steaks. Place oiled-side down on a hot barbecue and brush the tops with some more. If it looks like rain, pop them under a very hot grill (broiler). Cook for 4–5 minutes on each side.

Serve with bread and salad. Try a spoon of green caper or red onion relish on the side.

If you are lucky enough to find any of these magical and extraordinary creatures, choose a perfect unblemished one, carry it home gently and light the barbecue. They are common in pastures from mid to late summer and look like white footballs lost in the fields. One is usually more than enough for a family feast and they make wonderful soups and stews as well. If you are not lucky enough to find any, or if you are unsure about your mushroom identification skills, then try this with big and open flat field mushrooms (usually found in the supermarket).

MUSHROOMS À LA GRECQUE

6 tablespoons olive oil

12 tiny onions, peeled – the small pickling or red
    variety if you can, but it's still good without
    onions if you don't have any

4 cloves garlic, thinly sliced

2 teaspoons dried oregano

2 bay leaves

2 teaspoons coriander seeds

½ teaspoon dried thyme or 1 sprig fresh thyme

½ lemon, thinly sliced

1 teaspoon ground black pepper

Heat the oil in a pan until it is good and hot. Throw everything into the pan and shake and roll the ingredients about for about 8 minutes until the onions are beginning to brown. If you are not using onions, give it just 2–3 minutes.

350g (12oz/3 cups) whole small mushrooms

½ teaspoon paprika

Add to the pan and shake and turn for 2 minutes.

---

6 tablespoons organic white wine or white
    grape juice

3 tablespoons cider vinegar

juice of 1 lemon

4 tablespoons (¼ cup) water

2 tablespoons tamari soy sauce

Add to the pan and bubble madly for 3–4 minutes. Reduce the heat and simmer with the pan covered for 5 minutes. Leave to cool in the juices.

 Choose small, even, firm button mushrooms, or the brown chestnut variety.

Small pickling onions or red onions are best, but the mushrooms are still good without onions if you don't have any.

The flavour of this dish will develop gently if it is left to its own devices in the fridge for a couple of days.

MUSHROOM PERSILLADE WITH PASTA

8 tablespoons (½ cup) olive oil

6 cloves garlic, thinly sliced

100g (4oz/1⅓ cups) white mushrooms, thickly sliced

100g (4oz/1⅓ cups) chestnut mushrooms, thickly sliced

100g (4oz/1⅓ cups) oyster mushrooms, separated and cut in half if large

100g (4oz/1⅓ cups) fresh shiitake or ceps (porcini) sliced, or 50g (2oz/2 cups) dried mushrooms, soaked in hot water for 1 hour

Get the oil really hot in a large frying pan (a wok is best) and sizzle the garlic for a second before adding the mushrooms one type at a time. Stir and shake the mushrooms between each addition and let them squeak. Keep them really hot and moving for about 8 minutes.

1 teaspoon coarsely ground black pepper

a really big handful of chopped fresh parsley

3 tablespoons tamari soy sauce

a splash of red wine and/or a little of the water from the soaked mushrooms if you have it

2 tablespoons nutritional yeast flakes

Lower the heat a little and add to the mushrooms.

225g (8oz/2⅔ cups) pasta of your choice, cooked and drained

Stir well into the mushrooms and heat through.

 To serve, sprinkle with more parsley and yeast flakes. If you have a tiny bottle of truffle oil, drizzle 1 tablespoon on top before serving with a baby spinach leaf salad and garlic bread.

As with all the mushroom recipes, a combination of different types is best, but this dish will still taste delicious if you can only find the usual supermarket kind. Get them as they are just opening if you can.

I like to use a mixture of spinach and wholemeal (wholewheat) fusilli, but you can use whatever you have.

MAGIC MUSHROOM SOUP

*10 fresh shiitake mushrooms, sliced, or dried
    mushrooms, soaked until soft.*
10cm/4 inch piece of fresh root ginger, grated
1.8 litres (3 pints/7½ cups) water

Simmer together for 30 minutes. If using dried mushrooms, add the soaking water to the pot for extra flavour.

2–3 tablespoons organic miso paste, to your taste
6 spring onions (scallions), finely sliced

Add miso paste to taste and allow to melt gently for a few minutes. Do not boil. Add the onions (scallions) just before serving.

I feel that applying the word 'magic' to this reviving dish is justified – not only does it taste wonderful but it is also a great example of just how delicious combinations of healing foods can be. Because its effects are so remarkable I thought I would just list a few of its pharmacological workings:

- Shiitake mushrooms boost interferon levels and increase interleukin activity. They are also rich in polysaccharides.
- Ginger is rich in antioxidants and improves production of glutathione-s-transferase, a key enzyme responsible for detoxification.
- Mushrooms and garlic both support the immune system, balance hormone activity, improve liver function, inhibit damage to the DNA and excessive cell growth that can precede cancer.
- Organic miso is high in beneficial bacteria, and soya products are well known for their health support.

As well as all that it warms and cheers the spirit.

LENTIL AND GRAIN SOUP
WITH SEA VEGETABLES

1 onion, finely chopped *2 carrots, finely chopped* *1 potato, finely chopped* *2 celery stalks and a few leaves, chopped* *2 bay leaves* *4 tablespoons (¼ cup) olive oil*	Sauté together for about 10 minutes over a moderate heat until the onion is soft and transparent.
175g (6oz/scant 1 cup) barley *1.5 litres (2½ pints/1½ quarts) water* *2 tablespoons low-salt bouillon powder*	Add to the pan and bring to the boil. Reduce the heat and simmer for 30 minutes.
400g (14oz/2 cups) red lentils or yellow split peas *25g (1oz/heaping ½ cup) wakame seaweed* *juice of 1 lemon – optional*	Add to the pan and continue to simmer gently for 30 minutes until the lentils are beginning to break up.
2 sheets nori seaweed	Pop them under a hot grill (broiler) for a couple of seconds until they turn bright green. Crumble into crispy flakes and sprinkle on top of the soup.

 Mellow and warming.

A SOUP OF AGREEABLE ANARCHY

2 medium onions, finely chopped
2 medium carrots, finely chopped
4 cloves garlic, finely chopped
4 tablespoons (¼ cup) olive oil
1 tablespoon dried or fresh oregano
1 tablespoon dried or fresh basil

Sauté gently together in a nice big pan for 5 minutes. Lower the heat, cover and cook for 10 minutes.

3 tablespoons tomato paste
2 courgettes (zucchini), diced
100g (4oz/2 cups) cabbage, finely shredded
1 tablespoon low-salt bouillon powder
½ teaspoon ground black pepper
1 tablespoon tamari soy sauce

Stir the tomato paste into the softened onion mix and sizzle for a few minutes before adding the other ingredients. Stir and soften for about 10 minutes.

600ml (1 pint/2½ cups) tomato juice
25g (1oz/heaping ½ cup) dried wakame seaweed
1.2 litres (2 pints/5 cups) water

Stir into the pan and bring to the boil. Simmer gently for 40 minutes.

handful of fresh parsley or mixed herb leaves
1 tablespoon miso paste

Stir in and serve in big bowls.

 This soup gets its name from the fact that it's got just about everything in it. It's a very good first 'go' at sea vegetables because the flavour is very like the familiar minestrone and the sea flavour is very subtle. The taste develops overnight while the soup cools, and it goes on getting better and better with time, so make plenty. It will freeze well and you can add cooked grains or pasta to make it even more of a meal.

LIVE LEAVES

Shining, squeaking, singing dancing leaves – of all kinds – are absolutely essential in eating for health and energy. They are one of the richest sources of nutrients in the vegetable kingdom.

Their very greenness itself is good for us. The green pigment, chlorophyll, is very similar in its chemical structure to the hemoglobin in our blood and all leafy green vegetables are marvellous 'blood' tonics, especially helpful in cases of anaemia. Chlorophyll also has a remarkable ability to combine with toxins in the digestive system and remove them from the body.

Try to eat a wide variety of these wonder foods. Different plants, different shades of green, all have varying packages of nutrients to offer, but all contain beta carotene (vitamin A), vitamins B, C and E, iron, potassium, calcium, folic acid, minerals and trace elements.

It is worth noting the calcium. When first embarking on a new way of eating, many people have concerns about calcium. They are convinced that if they reduce or avoid milk and dairy produce they will become deficient in this vital mineral. A particular worry is over the formation of healthy bones and teeth in children. A moment's thought about where the cow gets its calcium from, the strength of its bones and teeth. The formation of the fantastic tusks of an entirely vegan elephant should start to put our minds at rest. They get it from eating leaves – and so can we.

Beware of always buying, cooking and eating the same leafy vegetables week after week throughout the year. Variety is as important as freshness, for both the nutrients and the flavour. Experiment with change – once you have tried a recipe and know that you have enjoyed it, try it using different leaves sometimes, and the more the better. I list a few here to encourage you.

Beetroot (beet) leaves
Brussels sprouts
Cabbage, of every description
Cavolo nero
Chinese leaves (Chinese cabbage)
Collard greens
Curly kale
Dandelion leaves
Kale
Mizuna greens
Nettle tops
Pak choi
Sorrel
Spinach
Spring greens
Swiss chard
Turnip tops
Watercress

Get them as fresh as you can – have fun – eat lots of leaves.

MAKE A MEAL OF LEAVES

1 tablespoon tamari soy sauce
2 tablespoons olive oil
juice of 1 lemon or lime
splash of cider vinegar
pinch of ground black pepper
1 teaspoon runny honey
2 teaspoons walnut oil – optional, but very good

Combine in a large bowl.

approximately 225g (8oz/1 cup) cooked beans –
*   flageolets or cannellini are best*
1 small red onion, very finely chopped
100g (4oz/1⅓ cups) firm white mushrooms, sliced

Gently stir into dressing and allow to marinate for 30 minutes. If the beans are still warm, let them cool in the dressing and then add the mushrooms later.

2 big handfuls of rocket (arugula) leaves

Mix in and serve immediately.

 If you are on your own for lunch, halve the quantities and eat the lot, otherwise this would be a good salad course for four.

SPINACH CHAPATIS

100g (4oz/¾ cup + 2 tablespoons) wholemeal
   (wholewheat) flour – attar or chapati flour if
   you have it
100g (4oz/2 cups) fresh spinach, very finely
   shredded
1 teaspoon onion seeds and/or sesame seeds
4 teaspoons tamari soy sauce
2 teaspoons water

Sift the flour on top of the spinach in a big bowl, then add everything else. Get both hands in the bowl and begin squeezing and kneading the flour into the spinach. For a few minutes this may seem a hopeless task, but keep on kneading with vigour … and keep on. Depending on your stamina, after about 10 minutes you will have a bright green and crumbly dough. Keep kneading and after a further 5 minutes you will have a speckled, bright green smooth dough. Wrap tightly in cling film (plastic wrap) and chill for at least 2 hours – it will keep happily in the fridge overnight.

Unwrap and roll the dough into a long sausage, divide into 8–10 pieces and roll each piece into a smooth ball. Sprinkle some flour on your board and rolling pin and roll each piece into a circle until it is about the thickness of a coin (as for pie crust). The pieces tend to stick, so keep them separate or flour them where they touch.

Heat a dry heavy pan or griddle until almost smoking and place a chapati in the middle. Cook for 3 minutes and then turn it over. It should begin to puff up a little bit as it cooks. Make a thick pad by folding a cloth, then press it down on the chapati a couple of times – this will encourage little bubbles of air to expand and lighten the finished bread. After 3–4 minutes of this, remove and wrap in a clean cloth while you do the others.

Pile the chapatis up as you go (they won't stick now) and keep warm. Dust any burnt flour specks from the pan between each one – do this carefully as it will be very hot.

On your first try you may find all this quite new but, as with any breadmaking, the more you do it the better it gets. Once you are confident, you will find that you can create a gentle rhythm by rolling one chapati and cooking another at the same time.

 Serve with little bowls of Kerala-style Spiced Cabbage (see page 74), Potatoes with White Poppy Seeds (see page 35) and some dhal, or just roll them up filled with a bean sprout salad and tahini.

BRUSSELS SPROUTS WITH NUTS AND LIME

1 tablespoon olive oil
1 small onion, very finely chopped
450g/1lb Brussels sprouts, each one cut
  into quarters
50g (2oz/scant ½ cup) pine kernels or almonds
grated zest (peel) and juice of 1 lime
pinch of ground black pepper
1 teaspoon malt extract
1 teaspoon tamari soy sauce – optional

Get the oil good and hot and toss everything into the pan. Stir and sizzle for a few minutes, then reduce the heat, cover and cook slowly for 15 minutes until soft.

 If you think you don't like Brussels sprouts, try them cooked this way.

CHOP SUEY

4 tablespoons (¼ cup) olive oil	Heat together in a big wok.
4 star anise	
1 tablespoon sesame oil	
5cm/2 inch piece of fresh root ginger, grated	

1 onion, sliced	Add to the wok, sizzle and stir until well mixed.
1 medium carrot, sliced	
1 small sweet green pepper (bell pepper), finely sliced	
1 teaspoon paprika	
1 teaspoon ground black pepper	

100g (4oz/1 cup) white button mushrooms, thickly sliced	Add to the wok, sizzle and stir until well mixed.

100g (4oz/2 cups) white or green cabbage, very finely shredded	Add to the wok, sizzle and stir until well mixed.
100g (4oz/2 cups) Chinese leaves (Chinese cabbage), less finely shredded	
225g (8oz/4 cups) pak choi, cut into 2.5cm/1 inch pieces, including the stems	

900ml (1½ pints/3¾ cups) water	In a big bowl, stir the water into the arrowroot or flour little at a time. Add to the vegetables with the tamari. Reduce the heat and cook gently for 5–10 minutes, until the vegetables are cooked to your taste.
2 tablespoons arrowroot powder, cornflour (cornstarch) or potato flour	
4 tablespoons (¼ cup) tamari soy sauce	

100g (4oz/heaping ½ cup) bean sprouts from mung beans or chick peas (garbanzo beans) *6 spring onions (scallions), shredded*	Scatter on top and serve with rice or noodles.

 Who knows where it comes from? China? America? Who cares – it's so good.

CAVOLO NERO WITH ROASTED FENNEL SEEDS

4 teaspoons fennel seeds *5 tablespoons olive oil* *2.5cm/1 inch piece of fresh root ginger, grated* *3 cloves garlic, grated* *1 green chilli, finely chopped* *½ teaspoon ground black pepper*	Roast the seeds for a few minutes in a wide heavy pan. Add the oil, heat and stir in the other ingredients. Stir over a high heat for a couple of minutes.
900g/2lb cavolo nero or dark green leaves, shredded	Throw handfuls of leaves into the pan and stir well before adding the next. Stir-fry for 6–7 minutes. Reduce the heat, cover and steam in their own juices until any stems are soft.
4 teaspoons tamari soy sauce – optional, to taste	Give the leaves a final few stirs over a high heat to get rid of any liquid, splash with the tamari and serve with grains.

 Cavolo nero is a wonderfully tasty kale that was most often seen in Italian cookery, but it is now becoming more widely available. Don't worry if you can't find any – you will also have great success with this recipe using kale, curly kale, spinach or chard leaves.

KERALA-STYLE SPICED CABBAGE

450g/1lb firm white or green cabbage,
    very finely shredded

3 tablespoons tamari soy sauce

Knead and scrunch together in a big bowl for 3–4 minutes to soften the cabbage. Set aside.

---

5 tablespoons olive oil

2 bay leaves

3 whole cloves

1 small stick of cinnamon

2 teaspoons whole cumin seeds

Heat together in a heavy pan until just smoking.

2.5cm/1 inch piece of fresh root ginger, grated

2 medium onions, finely sliced

Add to the pan and stir well. Lower the heat, cover and cook gently for 10 minutes until the onions are soft and slushy and are just going golden.

---

2 teaspoons turmeric

2 teaspoons ground coriander

½ teaspoon chilli powder – optional

Stir into the pan and cook over a low heat for 3–4 minutes. Add half the cabbage and stir well. Increase the heat, add the rest and stir over a high heat for 2–3 minutes. Cover tightly and continue to cook over a gentle heat for approximately 30 minutes. Give it a stir every 10 minutes or so, and add little splashes of water if it starts to stick. The cabbage should be really soft. Check for seasoning.

 So simple – so good. Try serving it with Ginger Brown Rice and Lentils (see page 84).

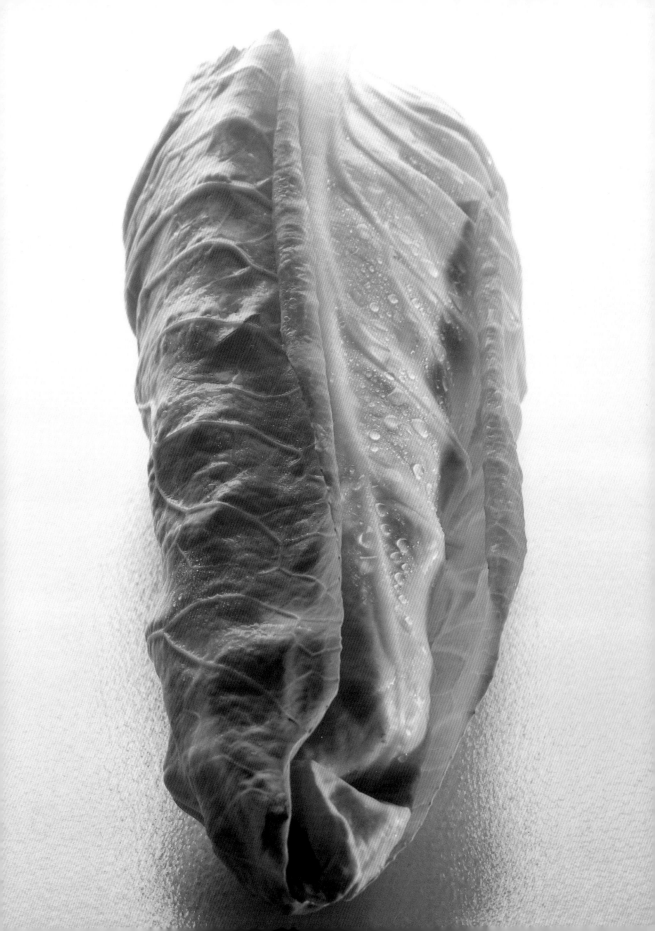

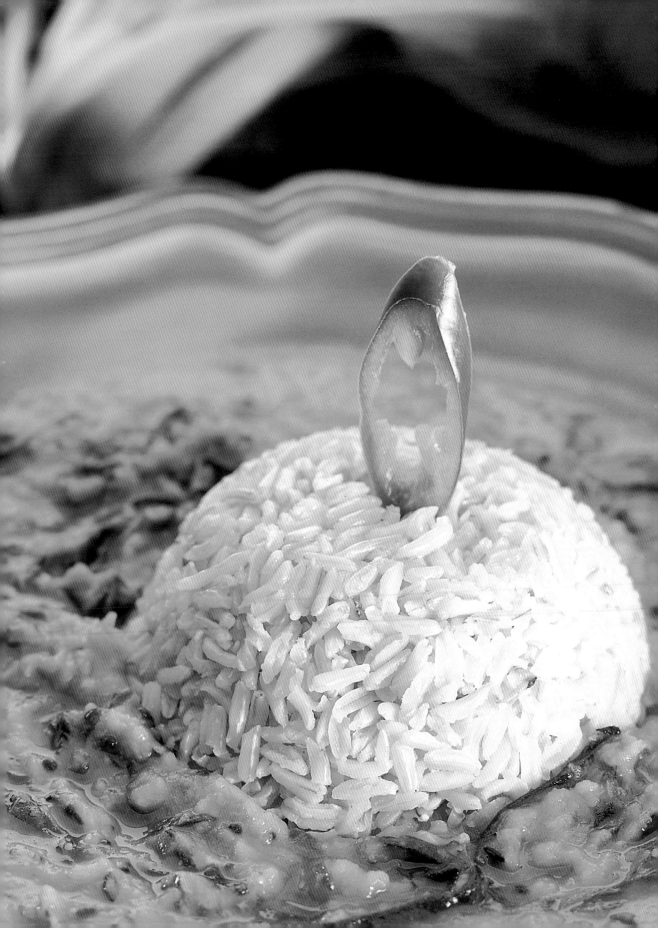

CHANNA DHAL WITH LEAVES

225g (8oz/1 cup) yellow split peas
1.2 litres (2 pints/5 cups) water
1 teaspoon low-salt bouillon powder – optional
1 teaspoon turmeric

Bring to the boil, reduce the heat to a gentle simmer, then partially cover and cook for 40 minutes until the lentils are soft. Keep the heat gentle as the water boils over easily and can make a real mess of your stove. When the lentils are soft, remove from the heat and give it a little whisk to break up some of the lentils.

2 tablespoons olive oil
2 bay leaves
1 teaspoon whole black mustard seeds
1 teaspoon whole cumin seeds
short stick of cinnamon
4 whole cloves

Heat the oil in a big heavy pan, add the bay leaves and spices and let them brown (to nearly burnt) and begin to smoke. Be confident here as the smoky taste is very good with lentils.

2.5cm/1 inch piece of fresh root ginger, grated
350g (12oz/6 cups) fresh spinach or chard leaves,
    roughly chopped and any tough stems removed

Quickly stir into your smoking pan, adding the ginger first. Watch out for spluttering. Stir to coat with the oil and spices. When the leaves have wilted down, pour in the lentils. The effect can be somewhat volcanic, so be careful and make sure you use a big pan. All this bubbling is worth it as it does combine the flavours wonderfully. Reduce the heat and simmer for 5 minutes to cook the leaves.

juice of 1 big lemon
1 small fresh green chilli, finely chopped – optional

Sprinkle on top just before serving.

 This dhal is rich and mellow. Try it served with rice or cooked grains, and Kerala-style Spiced Cabbage (opposite). If you want to serve it as a soup, add vegetable stock at the end.

CREAMY ONION GRATIN OF DARK GREEN LEAVES

OVEN: 190°C/375°F/GAS 5

approximately 1.4 kg/3lb curly kale, roughly chopped and tough stems discarded
8 cloves garlic, halved

Throw into a pan of boiling water, return to the boil and boil for 10 minutes. Drain well. The water is very good to drink or use in soup. Place the greens in an ovenproof dish so that it is about half full.

1 quantity Gentle Onion Sauce (see page 23)

Heat the sauce gently. Pour on top of the greens.

1 tablespoon olive oil
2 teaspoons tamari soy sauce
handful of poppy, sunflower, sesame and/or pumpkin seeds – optional

Sprinkle on top and bake in the oven for 20 minutes until browning and bubbling.

 A delightful way with any dark green vegetables or mixtures, but my favourite is curly kale or chard leaves and stems. The garlic is optional but don't be frightened of it, it will be sweet and mellow in the finished dish.

HILL STATION SPRING GREENS

1 tablespoon mustard oil – optional, look out for it
    in Asian stores
2 tablespoons olive oil
2 dried red chillies, whole
¼ teaspoon asafetida powder

Get the oils really hot, drop in the chillies and
asafetida, and sizzle for a second.

900g/2lb spring greens, shredded with tough
    stems removed
a few sprigs of fresh mint, roughly chopped
water

Add to the pan, stir-frying as you go. As the
greens start to wilt, splash in 3 tablespoons
water and reduce the heat, then cover and
cook very gently for 15 minutes.

tamari soy sauce – optional, to taste
very finely chopped fresh green chilli – optional

Sprinkle on top if you like. Serve with rice.

 It is only really in the mountainous areas of India that you see greens cooked in this simple style, as these loose-leaved vegetables need a little chill in the air to grow and they do not travel well. In cooler climates we are lucky enough to have them available most of the time.

Even by Indian standards this can be a very hot dish, so I have not included the amount of chilli that is traditional, and you can leave it out altogether if you like.

CURIOUSLY GREEN QUICHE

OVEN: 190°C/375°F/GAS 5

100g (4oz/1 cup) sesame seeds, roasted and ground
125g (4oz/¾ cup) wholemeal (wholewheat) flour
50g (2oz/½ cup) organic white flour
4 tablespoons (¼ cup) olive oil
1 tablespoon soya margarine
cold water, to mix

Combine the seeds and flours and rub in the fats. Sprinkle in just enough water to form a workable pastry. Knead gently for a couple of minutes and roll out. If it is a little bit sticky, or you are not having a very confident day, roll it between two sheets of floured cling film (plastic wrap). Use it to line a greased quiche pan, a 25cm/10 inch metal one with a loose base is best. Press it down well and chill.

6 or 8 green chard leaves, washed and stripped from the big white stems, or 900g/2lb spinach, washed and trimmed
2 tablespoons olive oil
2 cloves garlic, thinly sliced

If you are using chard, shred the stems and cook them in boiling water for 8 minutes. Drain and cool. If you are using spinach, just shred the leaves and sauté them in the oil and garlic for a couple of minutes, cover and simmer until soft and well cooked. Do the same with chard leaves.

100g (4oz/scant 1 cup) almonds

Whizz to a powder in a blender or food processor, then scatter half of the powder over your chilled pastry case.

225g (8oz/1 cup) plain silken tofu
½ teaspoon ground black pepper
½ teaspoon grated nutmeg
1 tablespoon nutritional yeast flakes – optional
juice of ½ lemon
2 tablespoons tamari soy sauce

Add to the almonds in the machine with either all the chard leaves or half of the spinach. Give the whole lot a quick blast, to blend. Spread the remaining spinach or the chard stems over the ground almonds on the pastry and pour your green cream on top. Bake in the oven for 35–40 minutes. Check it is not browning too fast and reduce the heat a little if it is. Allow to stand for 10 minutes and serve.

 I hope you can make easy sense of this as I have made it a 'two-in-one' recipe with options. Just to complicate things further it also works well with kale or watercress, but I leave any further adaptations to your own imagination.

This quiche is also good when served cold, when it will be a little firmer. If you prefer, you can bake the pastry blind first, but the almonds should ensure crispness.

GINGER BRAISED CABBAGE

1 tablespoon olive oil
5cm/2 inch piece of fresh root ginger, grated
approximately 750g/1½lb cabbage, finely shredded

Heat the oil in a heavy pan and throw in the ginger, stirring well as it will stick a bit. Keep the heat high and add the cabbage a handful at a time, stirring well between each addition. Stir and sizzle for 5 minutes for the cabbage to wilt. Reduce the heat, cover tightly and cook very gently for 25–30 minutes, stirring occasionally. If the cabbage starts to stick or burn, stir in a tablespoon of water.

 Use any very tightly packed firm cabbage – white, red, hispi, spring or basic green. A simple piece of alchemy.

This goes well with Winter Veggie Tarte Tatin (see page 32).

NO GRAIN ...
NO GAIN

One could almost say the more grain the more gain.

Grains are the seeds of various grasses containing all the vital life force to grow the plant – or us. Grains have been the main human fuel food for over 10,000 years, and they supply us with energy sustaining complex carbohydrates, proteins, B vitamins, vitamin E and many minerals – sometimes including the elusive selenium. They are also rich sources of starch and fibre.

A lack of fibre in our modern refined diets is thought to be a significant cause in the advance of many chronic, serious and deadly diseases. Even this alone should be reason enough to include many kinds of whole grain in our daily diets. As the fibre coverings of the grain are its vital life protection, so the fibre content of our foods can protect us against many ailments and safeguard our health.

There are a great variety of whole grains available and each is incredibly versatile, so it is delightful and easy to include them every day. If you doubt this, think of couscous and vegetable tagine on Monday, spinach chapatis on Tuesday, a pasta dish on Wednesday, date and malt tea loaf for tea on Thursday, bulgar salad on Friday, wholewheat toast for breakfast on Saturday and sticky 'not chocolate' and banana pudding on Sunday – and that is just from wheat. The list from rice would be endless too. Other grains to try and include are millet, barley, quinoa, oats and of course corn which, although we are accustomed to eating it fresh, also comes in the form of cornflour (cornstarch), cornmeal, polenta and popcorn.

There appears to be a lot of myth and mystery around the cooking of whole grains, with each culture developing methods to suit their way of life and nutritional needs. In general, use a heavy pot with a tight lid. Add the washed grain and water, bring to the boil and simmer gently, tightly covered, until the liquid is absorbed and the grains are tender. Soaking grains for at least an hour before cooking prevents too much cracking and consequent sticking, so if you like each grain separate this will do the trick. It will also mean that the water quantity and cooking time is a little less. Experiment and find your favourite ways for different dishes.

We need to ensure that we eat lots of dishes that include the actual whole grains in addition to all the things that are made from whole grains – such as breads, wholegrain pasta, crackers, tortillas, crêpes, pastries, cakes and cookies. Remember that any processing, even grinding to flour, will mean the loss of some nutrients, so have some of your grains absolutely whole at least once a day if you can.

Whole grains will pretty much keep forever as long as you protect them from moisture and bugs, but they do deteriorate more quickly once they are ground into flour or broken down, so buy these in amounts that you will use up more quickly.

As with the great family of beans, grains are fairly interchangeable in recipes and mixtures work well. If you have a sensitivity to gluten you should concentrate on millet, corn, rice, quinoa and buckwheat.

APPROXIMATE COOKING TIMES FOR GRAINS

FOR 225G (8OZ/1 CUP) DRY WEIGHT OF GRAIN.

GRAIN TYPE	WATER	SIMMERING TIME	APPROX YIELD
Barley	3 cups	1$\frac{1}{4}$ hours	3$\frac{1}{2}$ cups
Buckwheat	2 cups	15 minutes	2$\frac{1}{2}$ cups
Bulgar wheat, chewy	Soak in 4 cups hot water (to cover)	Drain after 30 minutes (no cooking)	2$\frac{1}{4}$ cups
Bulgar wheat, soft	2 cups	15 minutes	2$\frac{1}{2}$ cups
Couscous	Soak in 3 cups	Steam or bake 10 minutes	2$\frac{1}{4}$ cups
Millet	3 cups	35–40 minutes	3$\frac{1}{2}$ cups
Quinoa	2 cups	15 minutes	2$\frac{1}{2}$ cups
Rice, brown or basmati	1$\frac{1}{2}$ cups	25 minutes	2$\frac{1}{4}$ cups
Rice, brown – short or long grain	2 cups	45 minutes	3 cups
Wholewheat berries	3 cups	2 hours	2$\frac{1}{2}$ cups
Wild rice	3 cups	45–50 minutes	4 cups

BASMATI GREEN TERRINE

OVEN: 180°C/350°F/GAS 4

900g/2lb courgettes (zucchini), thinly sliced
2 teaspoons dried tarragon or
4 teaspoons chopped fresh tarragon leaves

Mix together and place in a colander or steamer over a pan of boiling water until soft and well cooked. Turn during cooking to make sure they are cooked evenly. Cool a little, then purée about two-thirds of the mixture through a sieve (strainer) or in a food processor or blender.

1 large onion, finely sliced
25g (1oz/2 tablespoons) soya margarine
1 tablespoon olive oil
450g/1lb spinach leaves, shredded

Sauté the onion in the fats until softening, then add the leaves and pepper. Stir well and sizzle until the spinach is cooked and the water has evaporated.

2 tablespoons nutritional yeast flakes
1 tablespoon tamari soy sauce
1 teaspoon ground black pepper

Stir into the spinach.

approximately 350g (12oz/2 cups) cooked brown
  basmati rice, or any brown rice you have
approximately 225g (8oz/1⅓ cups) cooked organic
  white basmati rice
olive oil, for brushing
2 tablespoons nutritional yeast flakes

Mix together and stir in half of the spinach and all of the courgette (zucchini) purée. Press half of this mixture into the bottom of a well-oiled casserole dish. Cover with the remaining vegetables and top with the rest of the rice. Smooth down and brush with olive oil. Sprinkle with the yeast flakes, cover and bake in the oven for 30 minutes. Uncover and brown with the heat increased to 200°C/400°F/Gas 6 for about 10 minutes.

This is a terrine in the old-fashioned sense of being baked in a deep ovenproof dish, traditionally earthenware, before serving with a spoon.

Try it with Red Onion Relish (see page 25) or Gentle Onion Sauce (see page 23).

GINGER BROWN RICE AND LENTILS

1 tablespoon olive oil
5cm/2 inch piece of fresh root ginger, grated

Heat together in a heavy pan.

200g (7oz/1 cup) brown basmati rice
200g (7oz/scant 1 cup) lentils or yellow split peas
water
2 teaspoons low-salt bouillon powder

Stir the rice and lentils into the ginger and add water to cover by about the depth of half your thumb. Throw in the bouillon powder, stir once and bring to the boil, then lower the heat, cover and simmer for 30–35 minutes (or 50 minutes in the oven at 190°C/375°F/Gas 5). All the water should be absorbed. Place a clean cloth or kitchen towel between the pan and the lid and leave for 5 minutes before serving.

 This is just the most wonderful, warming comfort food. You can use any kind of brown rice but it will take longer to cook than basmati (45 minutes), so add the lentils after 10 minutes or use whole green or brown lentils to start with. Serve with a sauce or green vegetables. Leftovers are very versatile – try some in Garlic Rice Galette (see page 121).

MULTIGRAIN MULTISEED BREAD

OVEN: 190°C/375°F/GAS 5

1 tablespoon dried yeast *5 tablespoons warm water*	Combine in a small jug and leave in a warm place until frothy. Leave for around 10 minutes.

2 tablespoons runny honey *2 tablespoons olive oil* *900ml (1½ pints/3¾ cups) warm water* *1 tablespoons tamari soy sauce – optional*	Combine with the yeast in a large mixing bowl.

900g (2lb/heaping 6 cups) strong wholemeal *(wholewheat) flour* *225g (8oz/1⅔ cups) strong organic white flour* *50g (2oz/⅓ cup) oats or oatmeal*	Sift into the bowl and mix well.

50g (2oz/⅓ cup) bulgar wheat, soaked in boiling *water for 15 minutes and drained* *50g (2oz/heaping ⅓ cup) millet, soaked in boiling* *water for 15 minutes and drained* *2 tablespoons black poppy seeds* *1 tablespoon linseed (flaxseed)* *2 teaspoons sesame seeds*	Add to the bowl and combine thoroughly. Turn on to a floured board and knead with floury hands for at least 10 minutes. Dust with flour if it seems sticky. You are aiming for a nice, pliable and elastic dough that will spring back when prodded.

6 tablespoons sunflower seeds

Sprinkle on the dough and continue to knead until the seeds are evenly mixed through. Form the dough into a neat ball and place in a lightly oiled bowl. Turn the dough once or twice so it has a coating of oil. Cover with a damp cloth and leave in a warm place until doubled in size – about 1–1½ hours.

Turn out on to a floured board and knead again for 5 minutes. Shape into three smooth oval loaves and place each on a baking (cookie) tray. Alternatively, you can bake them in a loaf pan or clean flowerpots – only half fill them at this stage. Leave the loaves in a warm place for about 40 minutes to double in size. Bake in the oven for 40–45 minutes.

 The bread with just about everything. These loaves keep or freeze well and will make a meal with soup or salad. You can substitute the weight of the soaked grains I have used for any leftover cooked grains – you can even use the porridge left from breakfast.

PERFECT PATTIES

1 quantity Ginger Brown Rice and Lentils (see page 84), cooled. This quantity will make 12–14 patties
2 medium onions, very finely chopped
handful of fresh coriander (cilantro), finely chopped
juice of ½ lemon
1 fresh green chilli, very finely chopped – optional
2 tablespoons tamari soy sauce
1 teaspoon ground black pepper

Mix together in a large bowl. Get your hands in and really knead the mix together so that it binds well.

50g (2oz/scant ½ cup) organic flour or wheat, rice or polenta meal, for dusting
olive oil, for frying

Divide the rice mixture into even amounts and form into balls. Place one on a floured surface and sprinkle the top with flour. Using two table knives or two narrow palette knives, pat down and rotate. This is very difficult to describe and very easy to do. It will make the patties look very neat and they will be easy to turn in the pan. Just keep patting the top down and pushing round with the other knife. Chill as you shape the others.

Fry for 5 minutes on each side in a little olive oil until crunchy and hot through.

 These are great served with vegetables or a sauce. Try them with the Red Onion Relish (see page 25). They also work well with salad in a sandwich or bun.

This is such a versatile method that I could probably fill a whole chapter with variations on the theme – I leave that to your own taste and imagination and give you the basics so that you have the idea to start you off. You can replace the coriander (cilantro) and chilli with pretty much anything that takes your fancy:

- sun-dried tomatoes and olives and a little tomato paste
- grated carrot and fresh tarragon leaves
- leftover curried vegetables
- corn kernels and parsley

SAGE AND ONION SAUSAGES

225g (8oz/heaping 1 cup) millet
100g (4oz/½ cup) buckwheat
900ml (1½ pints/3¾ cups) vegetable stock or
    water and low-salt bouillon powder

Simmer together until the grains are soft, about 15 minutes. Allow to cool.

2 medium onions, very finely chopped
3 tablespoons olive oil
2 cloves garlic, crushed
4 teaspoons chopped fresh or dried sage leaves
1 teaspoon thyme leaves
1 teaspoon ground black pepper

Cook gently in a heavy pan until the onions are soft, 10 minutes or so.

2 tablespoons tomato paste
1 tablespoon chopped fresh parsley
1 tablespoon toasted walnuts, finely chopped

Fry the tomato paste with the onions for a couple of minutes. Add the other ingredients and stir well. Tip on to the cool grains and knead until everything is quite firm and holding together.

2 tablespoons tamari soy sauce
6 tablespoons fine oatmeal, for coating
olive oil, for frying

Take about 2 tablespoons of the mixture and squeeze it into fat little sausage shapes. Pat them into a little fine oatmeal to coat. Repeat until you have about 24 sausages. Chill for 30 minutes. You can also wrap them individually and freeze them at this stage.

    Fry gently in a little oil until golden brown and hot through.

 These are lovely with braised roots and a green vegetable. They are also good with Gentle Onion Sauce (see page 23).

VEGETABLE BIRIANI

5cm/2 inch stick of cinnamon
6 cloves
4 cardamom pods
1 tablespooon whole cumin seeds
2 bay leaves
6 tablespoons olive oil
3 medium onions, finely grated
5cm/2 inch piece of fresh root ginger, grated
2 cloves garlic, grated

Heat the whole spices and the bay leaves in the oil until they are just smoking (the bay leaves will blacken). Throw in the other ingredients, stir for a few minutes and enjoy the smell, then reduce the heat. Cover tightly and cook gently for 10 minutes until the onions are soft and slushy.

3 medium potatoes, chopped into even bite-size pieces
2 medium carrots, diced small
1 small cauliflower cut into small florets, stems and leaves finely chopped

Stir into the onions over a gentle heat, replace the lid and cook for 5 minutes.

4 teaspoons tomato paste
2 teaspoons turmeric
2 teaspoons ground cumin
2 teaspoons ground coriander
juice of ½ lemon
3 tablespoons tamari soy sauce

Stir in a bowl to form a thick, smooth paste. Add to the vegetables, increase the heat and stir and sizzle for 5 minutes until the spices are well mixed and smelling good.

225g (8oz/1⅔ cups) shelled fresh peas and/or broad (fava) beans
225g (8oz/heaping 1 cup) brown basmati rice
water

Give the peas or beans and rice a good stir into the mix, cover them with water and give the pan a shake. The water should be 2.5cm/1 inch over the top of the goodies. Once boiling, cover tightly and reduce the heat to a very quiet simmer for 40 minutes (or place in a moderate oven at 180°C/350°F/Gas 4 for 45 minutes). The liquid should be fully absorbed and the vegetables soft.

MEDITERRANEAN MARVELS

Tomatoes, sweet (bell) peppers, aubergines (eggplants), garlic, basil, rosemary, oregano and olive oil, the common strand that binds them into a sumptuous whole is the warmth and energy of the sun, soaked up while they grow. To just think about them, cook them or eat them warms the soul and brings lightness to our being. The depth and flavour to provide the balance comes from the precious olive, growing on ancient small trees, the prolific fruit gives us rich, golden green oil. A monounsaturated oil and one of the best forms of fat in the diet. It can actually lower the levels of damaging cholesterol in our blood and protect against heart disease.

Although it can be a bit more expensive, the cold pressed, virgin or extra virgin oils are the best choice, both for flavour and because heat and chemicals have not been utilized in the extraction process.

This wonderful group of foods form part of the staple diet of many peoples from southern Europe right round to North Africa. The combination would seem to be a winner as in the areas where a traditional diet is eaten the incidence of cancer and heart disease are measurably lower. There is currently massive research into a nutrient, lycopene, available from tomatoes, and its effects on the prevention of and recovery from certain types of cancer. Fortunately this amazing antioxidant is still bioavailable even after cooking so eat, enjoy and be well.

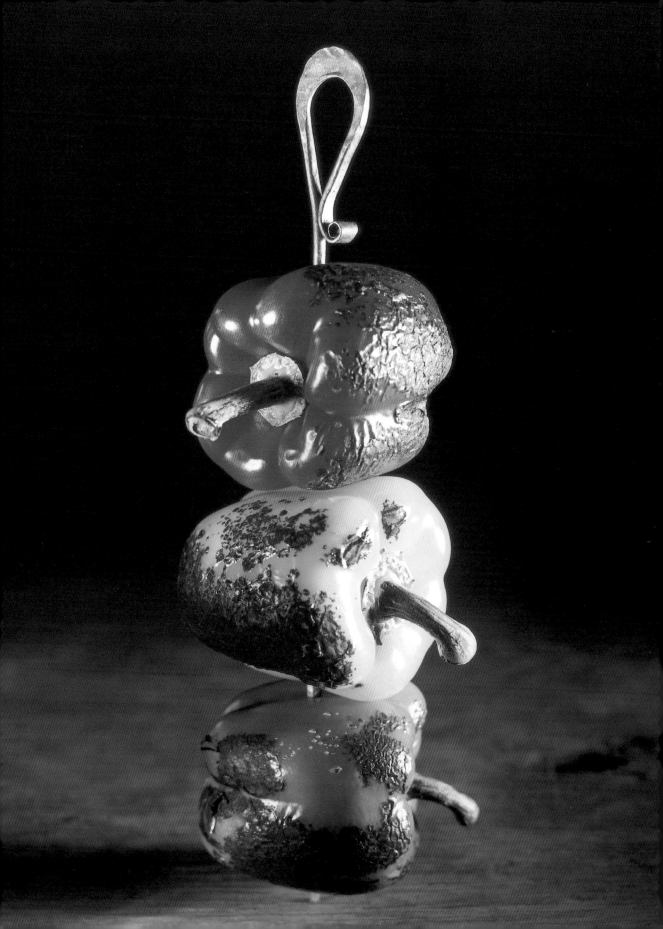

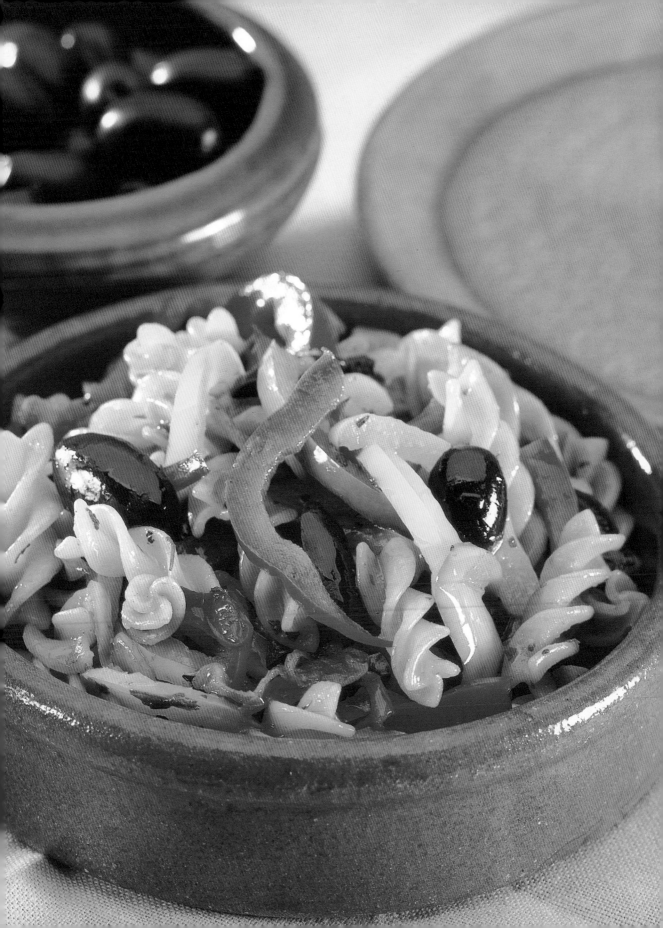

Modern Californian cuisine uses many of these sun-drenched foods with a flair unbound by tradition and with free, wild and delicious results. Free your soul, smell the basil and get sunshine into your kitchen.

RASTA PASTA

4 tablespoons (¼ cup) olive oil

2 teaspoons dried oregano

1 teaspoon dried basil

1 sweet red pepper (bell pepper), shredded

1 sweet green pepper (bell pepper), shredded

1 sweet yellow pepper (bell pepper), shredded

Heat the oil and herbs in a heavy pan, add the peppers and cook for a few minutes over a high heat until they begin to soften. Reduce the heat, cover and cook for 10 minutes.

225g (8oz/heaping 2½ cups) pasta, cooked

10 Kalamata black olives, stoned (pitted) and roughly chopped

Stir into the peppers and serve hot with the following sauce …

---

1 large sweet red pepper (bell pepper), roughly chopped

1 tablespoon olive oil

1 small sweet apple, chopped

1 tablespoon low-salt bouillon powder

450ml (15 fl oz/scant 2 cups) water

1 teaspoon low-salt yeast extract – optional

… cook the red pepper, oil and apple gently together in a separate pan for 8–10 minutes. Add the bouillon powder, water and yeast extract and simmer, covered, for 15 minutes until the pepper is very soft. Whizz in a blender or food processor until smooth.

Half wholemeal (wholewheat) and half spinach fusilli look very pretty.

Can also be served cold as a salad, with lots of chopped fresh parsley.

TOMATO SALAD WITH BLACK OLIVE DRESSING

8 luscious tomatoes, thinly sliced

2 small onions, thinly sliced and separated into rings

handful of fresh basil leaves, gently torn into pieces

Arrange in layers in a large shallow bowl.

150ml (5 fl oz/⅔ cup) olive oil

4 tablespoons (¼ cup) cider vinegar

1 clove garlic

½ teaspoon freshly ground black pepper

15–20 black olives – Kalamata have a good flavour

Remove the olive stones (pits). If you don't have a little tool for this, just bash each one (not too hard) with the bottom of a jar and you will then find it easy to remove the stone (pit). Pile all the ingredients into a blender or food processor and whizz. Pour on top of the salad and serve at room temperature.

A favourite stand-by for any day when tomatoes are sweet.

Don't be tempted by ready-stoned olives – they don't taste as good.

ROAST PEPPER SALAD WITH GREMOLATA

4 sweet peppers (bell peppers) – 2 red, 1 green and
*   1 yellow or orange*
olive oil, for drizzling

Blacken the whole peppers over a flame or under a very hot grill (broiler). Use long metal tongs or a skewer to turn them. They should be pretty evenly black all over. Drop them into a bowl of cold water and use both hands to slide off all the burnt skin. Rinse and split open (if they haven't split already), remove the seeds and spread flat on kitchen paper to dry. Arrange them on your most gorgeous serving plate and drizzle with olive oil to finish.

50g (2oz/1 cup) fresh parsley
2 cloves garlic, or more to your taste
grated zest (peel) of 1 orange
grated zest (peel) of 1 lemon

Make sure the parsley is nice and dry before you start and then tip on to a big chopping board and chop together until well mixed. I don't usually risk this in a food processor – you don't want to end up with a purée. Sprinkle on top of the peppers.

Serve on its own as a first course or with grilled (broiled) vegetables.

Gremolata is a vibrant seasoning and a colourful garnish that pops up in dishes all over Italy. The Milanese seem especially fond of it. Try it wherever you need that final burst of flavour.

TRIPLE TOMATO PESTO

12–15 sun-dried tomatoes in olive oil,
  roughly chopped
4 cloves garlic, chopped
50g (2oz/2 cups) fresh basil leaves, roughly
  chopped – more if you like
8 small ripe fresh tomatoes, roughly chopped
1 tablespoon tomato paste
2 teaspoons tamari soy sauce – optional
½ teaspoon ground black pepper
6 tablespoons olive oil, including the oil from
  the tomatoes
1 small fresh red chilli, chopped – optional

Don't waste the tasty oil from the sun-dried tomatoes, drain it into a bowl and use it instead of some of the olive oil. Put the ingredients in a food processor, one at a time in the order listed, pulsing to chop and mix well between each addition.

You will find many uses for this delicious pesto. To start you off, try it just stirred through cooked pasta, or mixed with cooked potatoes and grilled (broiled) until brown. It will enliven any sandwich and makes a lovely bruschetta topping.

 If you have not eaten it all at once, or if you make double, pesto will keep for about a week in a jar in the fridge as long as the surface is covered with a good layer of olive oil.

ROASTED MARVELS

OVEN: 220°C/425°F/GAS 7

4 good-size sweet red peppers (bell peppers), cut in half lengthways

First cut the peppers into halves – if you can manage to split the stems and leave half on each, it looks pretty. Take out the seeds and lay the pepper halves on their backs on an oiled baking (cookie) tray.

8 whole cherry tomatoes
4 whole cloves garlic
1 red onion, chopped
1 courgette (zucchini), very thinly sliced
2 tablespoons olive oil
2 tablespoons chopped fresh basil or oregano
1 teaspoon runny honey
1 teaspoon tamari soy sauce – optional
pinch of ground black pepper

Combine in a large bowl, using your hands to make sure everything is well covered in the juice. Distribute evenly into the waiting pepper halves and bake in the oven for about 20–30 minutes until the peppers are soft and collapsing but still holding all the goodies inside. They should be catching and browning on the top.

 Simple, juicy and dramatic.

Serve two each with a grain as a main dish, or one each with garlic bread as a first course. Transfer them carefully so you don't lose the juice.

SWEET, SOUR AND WARM CHATZILIM SALAD

OVEN: 200°C/400°F/GAS 6

*2 medium aubergines (eggplants), chopped
    into chunks*
6 tablespoons olive oil
2 teaspoons tamari soy sauce
1 clove garlic, crushed
1 teaspoon tomato paste

Combine well so that the pieces of aubergine (eggplant) are well covered. Lay them on a baking (cookie) tray and roast in the oven for 20 minutes. Leave them a little longer if they are not really soft and beginning to catch on the top corners.

juice of 2 lemons
1 tablespoon runny honey
pinch of ground black pepper
more crushed garlic, if you like
1 medium onion (red is pretty), very finely sliced
*2 handfuls of fresh parsley, broken up into
    small sprigs*

Mix well and add the hot aubergine (eggplant) pieces. If you are going to eat this cold add the parsley just before serving, otherwise just toss it all together and serve warm.

 I sometimes just cut everything much smaller and, once cooked pile on to slices of wholemeal (wholewheat) bread that have been brushed with garlic oil or basil oil and baked until crisp in a hot oven. To make sure everything is ready at the same time, do this when you cook the aubergines (eggplants). The crisp bread makes a wonderful little raft for soaking up the juices.

RUSTIC TUSCAN PIZZA

MAKES 1 LARGE OR 4 LITTLE INDIVIDUAL PIZZAS
OVEN: 230°C/450°F/GAS 8

1 tablespoon dried yeast
250ml (8 fl oz/1 cup) warm water

Mix in a large bowl and leave somewhere warm for 10 minutes until frothy.

350g (12oz/scant 2½ cups) strong wholemeal (wholewheat) flour, plus extra for kneading – you can use a mix of brown and white bread flours if you prefer
2 tablespoons olive oil
2 teaspoons tamari soy sauce

Mix into frothy yeast until you have a wettish dough. Turn out onto a well-floured surface and knead and stretch until you have a smooth elastic dough. You will need to knead for at least 10 minutes, adding more flour at the beginning as it will be sticky. Don't cheat on the time as this part really counts for good dough. Put the dough into an oiled bowl, cover with a damp cloth and leave in a warm place to double in size – about 1 hour.

Tip the dough back on to a floured surface and give it a few little punches, then knead again for a few minutes. Either roll and stretch into a big circle or divide into 4 balls and roll to make smaller bases. Place on an oiled baking (cookie) sheet and top with any of the following before baking in the oven for about 15 minutes.

* shredded spring onions (scallions) tossed in olive oil, tamari soy sauce, black pepper and nutritional yeast flakes.
* thinly sliced fresh tomatoes and onions tossed with olive oil, tamari soy sauce, chopped black olives, black pepper and oregano.

- spinach leaves and sliced onions sautéed in olive oil with garlic, tamari soy sauce and black pepper.
- thinly sliced mushrooms tossed with olive oil, rosemary, lemon zest (peel), sliced garlic, black pepper and tamari soy sauce.
- shredded sweet peppers (bell peppers) mixed with oil and hot chilli peppers if you like.
- any combination of the above.

The uncooked base can also be spread with a generous layer of Triple Tomato Pesto (see page 94) or tomato paste mixed with a little olive oil and herbs or garlic before adding any toppings. Alternatively, you can bake it with either of these tomato mixtures on their own and add no other toppings.

If you like something on the top as an alternative to cheese, try the following …

50g (2oz/¼ cup) plain silken tofu
3 tablespoons olive oil
2 cloves garlic
freshly ground black pepper
25g (1oz/⅔ cup) nutritional yeast flakes

… quickly blend together in a blender or food processor, scraping down the sides if it's reluctant to whizz, then dot over the topping 10 minutes into cooking.

HERB AND MUSTARD ROASTED EGGPLANT AND POTATO

OVEN: 190°C/375°F/GAS 5

450g/1lb new potatoes, thinly sliced

1 large aubergine (eggplant), cut into small cubes

3 tablespoons yellow mustard seeds, soaked overnight in cider vinegar, or 2 tablespoons Dijon mustard

2 tablespoons olive oil

1 tablespoon tamari soy sauce

2 cloves garlic, chopped – optional

1 teaspoon ground black pepper

Combine so that vegetables are well coated.

several sprigs of fresh herbs, such as thyme, rosemary and oregano, or 1 teaspoon each dried thyme, rosemary and oregano

Lay a large sheet of foil on the work surface and cover with a slightly smaller sheet of non-stick baking parchment. Lay half of the fresh herb sprigs on top, then tip on the vegetable mixture. Place the remaining herbs on top. Bring the long edges of the foil together and fold to seal, then fold in the short ends to make a flat neat parcel that is completely sealed. Carefully place it on a baking (cookie) tray and bake in the oven for 1 hour.

Unwrap very carefully and slide off the paper into a shallow ovenproof dish, removing some of the sprigs as you go. Pop under a hot grill (broiler) to crisp up a bit more if you like, or serve it as it is with a sprinkle of greenery.

 As usual, I am giving you one idea for this dish to start you off. Try other combinations cooked in this way. This one is also delicious with the addition of a few cooked beans.

CREAMED GARLIC DIP/SAUCE/SOUP

50g (2oz/1 very thick slice) wholemeal
   (wholewheat) bread, soaked in soya milk
175g (6oz/2 cups) almonds, ground
6 large cloves garlic, peeled – more if you
   can take it
2 teaspoons tamari soy sauce
½ teaspoon ground black pepper
½ teaspoon ground coriander – optional
8 tablespoons (½ cup) olive oil

Squeeze any liquid from the bread. Put everything apart from the oil into a food processor with a sharp blade and blend until there are no lumps of garlic to frighten the unsuspecting. Slowly add the oil while still whizzing – as you would for mayonnaise. Depending on how you want to serve this sauce, you can vary the thickness by adding cold water or soya milk.

 Known as *skordalia* in Greece, there is a local version of this sauce in almost all of the Mediterranean countries – it is renowned for preventing colds and infections. Try it thick with grilled (broiled) vegetables, or blend it until thinner and serve as a chilled soup with crisp romaine or Cos lettuce leaves and wholemeal (wholewheat) toast.

If you have the time and inclination you can remove the almond skins first. This will make everything that little bit paler and smoother. To do this, drop the almonds into boiling water, remove from the heat and leave for 10 minutes. Rinse in cold water and the skins should slip off easily.

GOLDEN TOFU PAELLA

OVEN: 180°C/350°F/GAS 4

8 tablespoons (½ cup) olive oil
2 medium onions, chopped
2 bay leaves
4 cloves garlic, sliced

Soften together for 5 minutes in a heavy pan with an ovenproof lid.

---

1 tablespoon turmeric
350g (12oz/2 cups) firm tofu in bite-size cubes, previously frozen and thawed in boiling water – see page 135
225g (8oz/2⅔ cups) fresh green beans (French/bobby), cut in half
225g (8oz/heaping 1 cup) fresh corn kernels cut from the cob
1 large sweet red pepper (bell pepper), cut into thin strips

Stir the turmeric into the onions and cook over a high heat for 2 minutes before adding everything else. Stir gently to make sure the onions are mixed through.

100g (4oz/heaping ½ cup) brown rice
100g (4oz/heaping ½ cup) organic white basmati rice
juice of 1 lemon
½ lemon, thinly sliced
water

Stir in with enough water to cover by about 2.5cm/1 inch. Bring to a gentle boil, cover tightly and place in the oven for 45 minutes. Alternatively, simmer very gently on top of the stove, but you will need to check it doesn't burn and you may need to add a little more liquid.

 Serve with lemon wedges, chopped fresh basil, shredded spring onions (scallions) or chopped fresh parsley and a salad.

CREAMY VEGETABLE RISOTTO

1 medium onion, finely chopped

1 large carrot, finely chopped

100g (4oz/1⅓ cups) firm mushrooms,
   finely chopped

2 courgettes (zucchini), finely chopped

5 tablespoons olive oil

2 bay leaves

1 tablespoon dried basil

1 small aubergine (eggplant), finely chopped

Make sure all the vegetables are cut into tiny pieces. Sauté everything together gently in a heavy pan for a few minutes.

350g (12oz/heaping 1½ cups) brown rice

50g (2oz/⅓ cup) wild rice – optional

2 tablespoons low-salt bouillon powder

900ml (1½ pints/3¾ cups) water to cover by
   2.5cm/1 inch

Stir the rice into the vegetables and add the bouillon powder and water. Bring to the boil, lower the heat and cover, then simmer until the rice is soft and the liquid absorbed, approximately 35 minutes. Remove from the heat and place a clean cloth or kitchen towel between the pan and the lid to absorb the steam and to fluff up the rice.

50g (2oz/¼ cup) plain silken tofu

2 tablespoons tamari soy sauce

1 teaspoon ground black pepper

2 tablespoons soya milk

Whizz together in a blender or food processor until smooth, then stir gently into the rice and heat through.

---

3 tablespoons nutritional yeast flakes

3 tablespoons chopped fresh parsley

Tip the rice into a warm serving dish and sprinkle the yeast flakes and parsley on top.

 This is very good with Basil and Garlic Roasted Red Roots (see page 26).

TUSCAN POLENTA

1.2 litres (2 pints/5 cups) water
1 clove garlic, finely chopped
450g (1lb/3 cups) polenta

Bring the water and garlic to the boil and pour in the polenta in a steady stream, stirring continually. Lower the heat and continue to stir until you have a smooth fluffy paste. This can take 10–35 minutes depending on the coarseness of your polenta. Taste a little to be sure it doesn't have a hard grainy texture. It will be smooth when cooked and quite stiff. Remove from the heat.

225g (8oz/1 cup) sun-dried tomatoes in olive oil, chopped.
2 tablespoons vegan pesto or chopped fresh basil leaves with 1 tablespoon olive oil
½ teaspoon ground black pepper
1 tablespoon tamari soy sauce
2 tablespoons finely chopped fresh parsley
2 teaspoons finely chopped fresh oregano, if you have any

Stir frantically into the polenta until well mixed. You can serve the dish at this stage with a tomato and onion salad, or it is also nice served instead of mash. Alternatively, tip the lot into a loaf pan lined with oiled-cling film (plastic wrap) or greaseproof (waxed) paper, cover and chill. It will happily wait in the fridge overnight. Cut into slices about as thick as your finger and then cut them diagonally. The shape is up to you – you can make them look pretty by using pastry (cookie) cutters. Brush the slices with oil and crisp on a hot griddle, or in a heavy frying pan with a little oil, or in a hot oven.

 Serve with sauce/salsa/salad or piled with Ginger Braised Cabbage (see page 79). Halve the quantities for a first course with salad.

TUNISIAN-STYLE ONIONS AND QUINOA

450g (1lb/2 cups) quinoa
double the volume of water

Bring the water to the boil and add the grain. Return to the boil and reduce the heat to a simmer. Cover tightly and cook gently for 15 minutes. Switch the heat off and leave covered for 5 minutes.

4 onions, finely sliced
4 cloves garlic, thinly sliced – optional
6 tablespoons olive oil
1 teaspoon whole coriander seeds

Take a separate pan and cook gently together for 5 minutes until the onions are softening.

2½ tablespoons tomato paste
4 tablespoons currants or raisins, or a mixture
½ teaspoon ground black pepper

Stir into the onions and continue to cook gently, stirring, for about 10 minutes.
     Mix thoroughly into the quinoa.

 Sprinkle with lots of fresh coriander (cilantro) leaves or flat-leaf parsley and serve as a grain accompaniment. Try it with Roasted Marvels (see page 95).

ROARING RAW POWER

When it comes to repairing, regaining and maintaining your health, raw foods are the business. They will supply you with more vitamins and minerals than you gain from cooked foods, they help eliminate toxins, and they will strengthen and support your immune functions. As you increase the amounts of fruit and vegetables you eat raw, you will quickly notice an increase in your vitality and an improvement in the way your skin glows and your body feels.

For some reason the word 'raw' can sound a little uninspiring, yet when you try some of the recipes in this section I am sure you will realize that this part of our diet can give us not only energy and health but delicious delight too.

It is such a pleasure to be able to talk about eating foods in abundance because much of nutrition these days is about the 'don'ts' rather than the 'dos'. With raw food there are really no reservations, and by including more and more you will find that you naturally cut back on some of the less positive aspects of your diet.

For best health aim to include salad, juice or fruits at least three times a day – eg fresh juice with breakfast, a big salad at lunch (it can be in a sandwich) and a salad or fruit salad in the evening as a first course, side dish or dessert.

It is often the wonder of dressings that can make the difference between enjoying salads or not. They are also a good place to redress the fat balance of a meal. For instance, if you have planned to include a pastry dish as part of the meal, which is comparatively high in fat (to be edible I feel pastry must have at least half fat to flour), then try an oil-free dressing on the salad. Timing counts, so remember to prepare the salad just before you eat – salad that has been sitting around after preparation runs the risk of becoming a bowl full of plant fibre with much of the nutrient value lost. Use dressings containing oils at room temperature – they will spread further and taste better.

Creating cocktails of fruit and vegetable juices can be a good way of obtaining the nutrients they have to offer in a pure and concentrated form. They are especially useful if your appetite is decreased due to illness or treatments, if your spirit is low and you need revitalizing, or if you are on a temporary detox or weight-loss programme. I have included just a few combinations in this chapter to get you in the mood – there is no doubt that regular fresh juices will improve your health and zest for life.

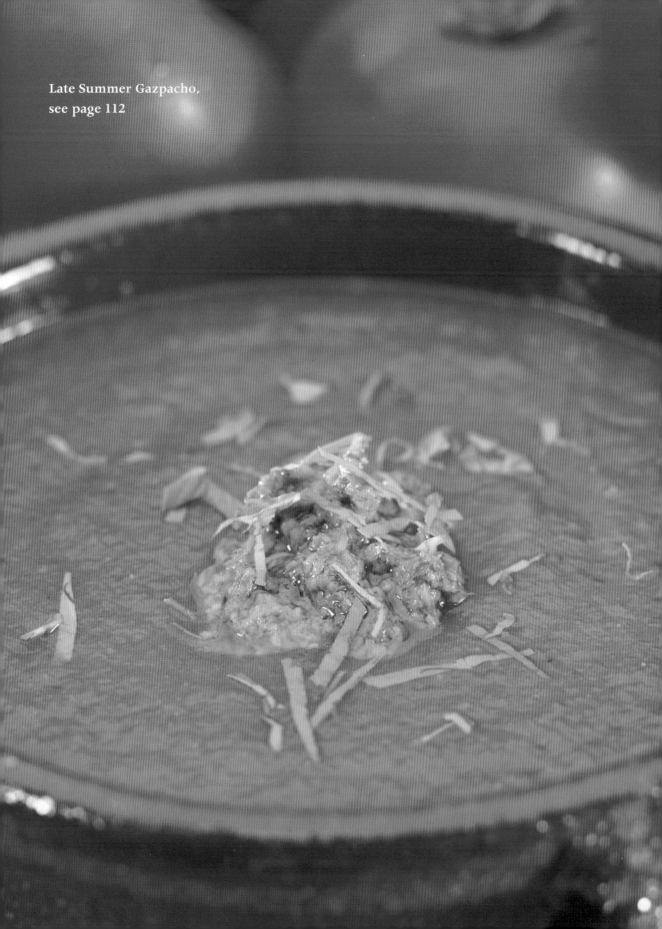

Late Summer Gazpacho,
see page 112

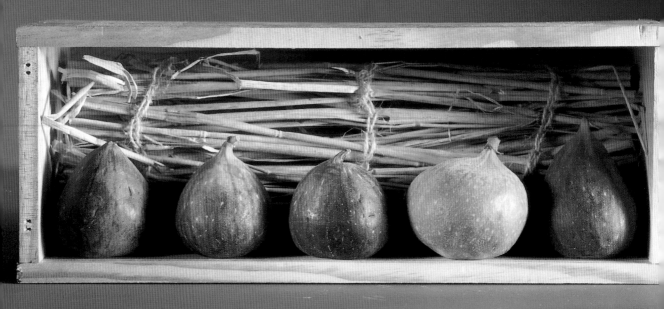

LAVISH AND LOVELY FRUIT SALAD

1 small sweet melon, such as charentais, ogen or
    honeydew, cut into small pieces
8 fresh lychees, peeled, pipped and halved
2 ripe kiwi fruit, peeled, halved and thinly sliced
2 handfuls of sweet seedless grapes, halved
2 ripe pears, cut into tiny cubes
juice of 1 orange
2 sweet, ripe fresh figs, thinly sliced (optional)

Mix gently together in a pretty bowl.

225g (8oz/1⅔ cups) ripe strawberries, or 1 ripe
    mango, or 225g (8oz/2 cups) raspberries
2 tablespoons maple syrup – optional
juice of 1 lemon or lime

If you are using a mango, peel it thinly and cut and squeeze the flesh from the stone (pit). Put the fruits, the juice and the syrup (if using) into a blender or food processor and whizz until smooth. Pour over the fruit salad, mix carefully and leave to stand for 10 minutes before serving – if you can wait.

 I have used a favourite combination, but do try different mixtures of your own. This is one to get addicted to.

A FRISSON OF FRISÉE

approximately 225g (8oz/2⅔ cups) curly endive
   (chicory) leaves, washed and bitter dark green
   part discarded
approximately 225g (8oz/2⅔ cups) radicchio
   leaves, washed and trimmed
100g (4oz/1 cup) walnut pieces, toasted in a dry
   pan for about 5 minutes

Gently break the leaves into bite-size pieces
and combine with the walnuts.

2 tablespoons walnut oil
1 tablespoon olive oil
1 tablespoon balsamic vinegar
1 tablespoon fresh orange juice
1 tablespoon tamari soy sauce
pinch of ground black pepper
1 teaspoon runny honey

Combine and drizzle over the salad. Enjoy
immediately as a first course or side dish.

 Curly endive (chicory), called *frisée* in French, is a beautiful being – a mass of curling green and
cream leaves with a juicy edge to the flavour. The greener leaves have a slight bitterness, so make
sure you choose one with a really creamy yellow or white blanched heart. You also see it ready
prepared in bags, but of course any salad that you buy already cut will have lost many of its
nutrients.

The lovely glowing radicchio matures in the same season, so it is a natural member of the same
family to mix in with this salad, so too is the fat white bud of whitloof chicory (Belgian endive).

CUCUMBER IN A CREAMY MINT DRESSING

½ cucumber, peeled and chopped
175g (6oz/¾ cup) plain silken tofu
grated zest (peel) of ½ lemon
juice of 2 lemons
2 teaspoons light tahini
2 teaspoons cider vinegar
½ teaspoon ground black pepper
handful of fresh mint leaves or 2 teaspoons
    dried mint

Whizz until smooth in a blender or food processor.

1 large cucumber, grated or thinly sliced
fresh mint sprigs

Mix the cucumber into the dressing and garnish with mint sprigs to serve.

 Apart from being refreshing and tasty, this is a good example of the way in which protein comes in unexpected forms in this style of healthy eating. Here, it is in the dressing.

FRESH MANGO SALSA

1 medium onion, chopped
1 fresh green chilli, chopped.
100g (4oz/2 cups) fresh coriander (cilantro),
  chopped
1 sprig of fresh mint – optional
1 teaspoon runny honey
juice of 1 lemon
pinch of ground black pepper
pinch of paprika

Pile into a food processor with a sharp blade and pulse a few times to an even texture but not a smooth purée.

1 large ripe mango

Peel the mango carefully, remove the flesh from the stone (seed) and chop into tiny pieces. Stir into the onion mixture and chill before serving.

 The texture of a good salsa should be somewhere between a sauce and a finely chopped salad, and this one has a delicious fresh zing. If you don't want the heat, use $1/2$ sweet green pepper (bell pepper) instead of the chilli.

Good in a tortilla with chilli beans and shredded lettuce or with Onion and Potato Pakoras (see page 36).

GIANT RADISH RÉMOULADE

20–25cm/8–10 inch white radish (mooli) cut into
    julienne strips (fine matchsticks)
1 medium carrot, grated
85g (3oz/⅔ cup) celeriac (celery root), peeled and
    cut into julienne strips
juice of 1 lemon

Mix gently together.

225g (8oz/1 cup) plain silken tofu
3 tablespoons cider vinegar
2 tablespoons olive oil
1 tablespoon tamari soy sauce
½ teaspoon ground black pepper
2 tablespoons Dijon mustard

Whizz until smooth in a blender or food
processor.

2 tablespoons pickled gherkins or dill pickles, very
    finely chopped
2 tablespoons finely chopped fresh parsley

Mix into the vegetables with the mayonnaise.
Serve as a salad or on mixed green leaves as a
first course.

The tofu mayonnaise is delicious and works well with different combinations of raw vegetables,
or simply as the 'mayo' in a sandwich.

If you can get organic Dijon mustard it has a great flavour, but it is much hotter, so taste as you go.

LATE SUMMER GAZPACHO

12 ripe tomatoes, chopped

2 cloves garlic

1 medium sweet red pepper (bell pepper), chopped

2 celery stalks, thinly sliced

1 teaspoon tomato paste

1 teaspoon paprika

pinch of ground black pepper

1 tablespoon tamari soy sauce – optional

½ lemon, sliced

1 tablespoon cider vinegar

Whizz in a blender or food processor until smooth, then pour through a sieve (strainer), pushing it through with the back of a ladle into a bowl. Any bits left in the sieve can go in a stockpot if you have one on the go. Chill in the fridge.

25g (1oz/½ cup) soft fresh bread, no crusts

50g (2oz/scant ½ cup) almonds or pine kernels, lightly toasted in a dry pan

3 cloves garlic – or more to your taste

grated zest (peel) of 1 lemon

2 teaspoons tamari soy sauce – optional

pinch of ground black pepper

Pulse to a rough paste in a food processor with the sharp blade, starting with the crumbs, nuts and garlic.

100g (4oz/2 cups) fresh rocket (arugula) leaves

Add the leaves to the processor, keeping behind a few sprigs. Whizz until well mixed.

4 tablespoons (¼ cup) olive oil

Pour in a steady stream while still whizzing.

Allow the pesto to stand for a few minutes while you pour the soup into individual serving bowls – nice wide shallow ones if you have them. If you have an extra tomato, place a thick slice in the middle of the soup and top with a good spoon of the pesto. Garnish each serving with a tiny sprig of rocket (arugula) and serve with warm bread. Serve extra pesto separately to spread on bread, or keep it for sandwiches.

Feel free to have this at any time of the year, but late, ripe, sweet summer tomatoes add a magical depth of flavour. Whenever you make it, choose the tastiest tomatoes you can find.

There are many variations of this chilled soup to be found in the different regions of Spain. This one from Andalusia is often served with a little mound of tasty extras in the middle of the dish or on the side. It makes a lovely summer first course.

If you choose, you can do the first part through the juicer for a lovely 'Virgin Mary' cocktail.

MISTO MISO PESTO

50g (2oz/1 cup) fresh parsley, roughly chopped

100g (4oz/2 cups) young spinach leaves, shredded

100g (4oz/2 cups) fresh basil leaves, roughly chopped

175g (6oz/heaping 1 cup) pine kernels or almonds

6 cloves garlic, sliced

pinch of ground black pepper

Pile into a food processor with a sharp blade and pulse a few times to mix, then whizz to a rough purée.

2 heaped tablespoons miso paste – barley miso is very good in this recipe but any variety will be fine

6 tablespoons olive oil

Add the miso and pour in the olive oil while the mix whizzes.

 A fine mix of raw greenery that packs a punch of flavour into dressings, grains, pasta or just on hot toast.

If you don't eat it all at once this will keep happily in a jar in the fridge for a few days.

PERFECTLY PINK SALAD – EXCEPT FOR THE ORANGE

450g/1lb red cabbage, very finely shredded
1 tablespoon tamari soy sauce
1 tablespoon cider vinegar

Place in a large bowl and scrunch and knead together with your hand for a few minutes. Set aside.

2 raw or cooked apple-size beetroots (beets), peeled and grated
grated zest (peel) of 1 orange
2 large oranges, skin and pith removed and flesh sliced
10–12 radishes, grated or thinly sliced
2 tablespoons olive oil – optional
½ teaspoon ground black pepper

Gently combine with the cabbage and allow to stand for a few minutes before serving.

 You can serve this on a bed of mixed green leaves, but it looks really stunning on the glossy pink of radicchio.

ROASTED SEED AND CARROT SALAD

450g/1lb carrots, grated

grated zest (peel) and juice of 1 lime

2 tablespoons fresh coriander (cilantro), parsley or
  mint leaves, or a mixture if you like, finely
  chopped

Combine in a serving bowl.

---

2 tablespoons olive oil

1 teaspoon whole black mustard seeds

½ teaspoon asafedita powder

2 teaspoons cumin seeds

2 teaspoons sesame seeds

2 teaspoons sunflower seeds

1 dried red chilli, chopped – optional

Heat the oil in a heavy pan. When it is very hot, throw everything in and sizzle and pop for a few seconds, then reduce the heat a little while the sunflower seeds go golden. Tip into the bowl of carrots, mix and serve.

SALAD OR JUICE - IT'S A TONIC

2 medium raw beetroot (beets), peeled and grated

3 medium carrots, scrubbed or peeled and grated

½ cucumber, thinly sliced

2 sweet apples, grated

grated zest (peel) and juice of 1 large orange

2 tablespoons chopped fresh parsley

1 tablespoon chopped fresh mint leaves

Combine in a bowl, or juice and drink immediately.

1 teaspoon runny honey – optional

1 teaspoon walnut oil – optional

1 teaspoon tamari soy sauce – optional

½ teaspoon ground black pepper

2 tablespoons toasted walnuts, chopped

Mix and sprinkle over the salad to serve.

This is a real power-packing combination – a real restorative for energy and a blood builder, recommended if you suffer from anaemia, great if you are pregnant and good for that 'time of the month'.

If you are not in the mood for salad, just push all the vegetables, fruit and herbs through the juicer. The salad's also very good in a sandwich or pitta bread with tahini.

CHINESE LEAVES WITH MISO DRESSING

2 tablespoons miso paste

4 tablespoons (¼ cup) light tahini paste

2 tablespoons cider vinegar

1 teaspoon malt extract (malt syrup)

pinch of ground black pepper

about 4 tablespoons (¼ cup) water

Combine in a little bowl or jug to make a smooth runny cream. Add a little water as you go to get it just right.

1 firm head Chinese leaves (Chinese cabbage), very finely shredded

Pile into a bowl and pour the dressing over just as you serve.

 Sprinkle with some sesame seeds if you have some.

Miso dressing livens up any bowl of raw veggies that you happen to have.

SQUASH FOR ALL SEASONS

I have given this mighty family of vegetables a chapter of its own as the chances are that at any given time of the year you will have at least one of its members in your kitchen. There are some 800 species in this group, known collectively as the 'cucurbita' family. Buying them can be a bit confusing as often the same variety seems to be known by many different names. If you buy in a supermarket, squash will most likely be called by their North American names, whereas when you buy them in ethnic stores they may have an Oriental or Caribbean name. Strangely, some of the most tasty seem to be known by their Japanese names.

With all vegetables, their seasonal freshness is important for your nutrition, so perhaps it is most useful not to worry about individual names but to simply divide them into summer or winter squash. The nutrients vary considerably, but all can taste fantastic. In general they are all low in calories and a good source of starch and fibre, and they will contain varying amounts of protein, vitamin A (beta carotene), folic acid, potassium, B vitamins, iron, calcium, vitamin C and sulphur. Summer squash are best eaten fresh and do not store well. They are thin-skinned and taste good when eaten raw if they are young and still have soft seeds. Their flavours are usually light and refreshing. Green or golden courgettes (zucchini), marrow (vegetable marrow), cucumber, golden nugget, crookneck, Little Gem, vegetable spaghetti and patty pan are all summer squash.

Winter squashes can be eaten young, but they have the advantage of storing well and continue to develop flavour late into winter. They have hard seeds and thicker skins than the summer squash. Their texture is firmer and less watery and their flavours are rich and satisfying. Most winter squash are generally interchangeable in recipes, but each does have its particular strengths that can make all the difference. The small ones, like tiny acorn, Delicata and Lady Godiva, are perfect individual 'stuffers'. The bigger, orange-fleshed varieties, such as Sweet Mama, kabocha, Hubbard, Turk's Turban and butternut, are luxuriant with flavour and good for roasting and using in soups.

The often giant, orange-skinned pumpkin has a lighter taste and texture and extremely nutritious seeds. If anyone in your home wants something to do while you are cooking pumpkin, give them the seeds and a bowl of warm water. Get them to wash away all the slippery strings and spread the seeds on a towel or kitchen paper to dry, then toast them on a baking (cookie) sheet in the oven until crisp. They're delicious to nibble and high in protein, zinc and minerals.

GARLIC RICE GALETTE

5 medium courgettes (zucchini), thinly sliced

8 cloves garlic, sliced

6 tablespoons olive oil

½ teaspoon ground black pepper

8 sweet fresh tomatoes, roughly chopped – skin them first if you prefer

1 tablespoon tomato paste

Toss together over a high heat, adding the tomatoes and tomato paste when the courgettes (zucchini) are just beginning to brown. Sizzle wildly for 3 minutes, then reduce the heat and simmer gently, covered, for 15 minutes. Set aside.

2 tablespoons olive oil

1 tablespoon tamari soy sauce

625g (1¼lb/3⅓ cups) cooked brown rice, or any mixture of cooked grains such as Ginger Brown Rice and Lentils (see page 84)

2 cloves garlic, crushed

Line a loose-bottomed 30cm/10 inch cake pan or large flan dish with non-stick paper and brush well with the oil and tamari. Take a couple of large spoonfuls of the courgettes (zucchini) and mix into the rice with the crushed garlic. Press half into the bottom of the cake pan. Spread the rest of the courgette (zucchini) mixture over it, leaving about 1cm/½ inch clear around the edge. Place the rest of the rice over the top a spoonful at a time, starting round the edge and smoothing in towards the middle. Press down gently and seal well with the back of a wet spoon. Brush with oil and bake in the oven for 25 minutes until golden and crunchy on top. Remove from the oven and leave to stand for 5 minutes. Cover with a large serving plate and invert, carefully remove the pan and paper and serve hot.

LAYERED MARROW GRATIN

OVEN: 180°C/350°F/GAS 4

6 tablespoons olive oil 2 large onions, finely chopped 6 cloves garlic, roughly chopped 2 teaspoons dried basil 2 teaspoons dried oregano or a handful of fresh oregano	Sauté together in a large heavy pan until the onions are soft, mushy and transparent.
4 heaped tablespoons (heaping ¼ cup) tomato paste	Add to the onion mixture and stir well over a low heat for about 5 minutes until the oil is separating.
450g (1lb/2⅔ cups) cooked aduki or red kidney beans 8 fresh tomatoes, chopped, or 2 x 400g/14oz cans 300ml (10 fl oz/1¼ cups) water 2 tablespoons tamari soy sauce 1 teaspoon ground black pepper 1 tablespoon low-salt bouillon powder	Add to the pan, stir well and cook gently, uncovered, for 35–40 minutes. Keep an eye on it as it cooks. It should become quite thick and reduced, so beware it doesn't stick.
85g (3oz/6 tablespoons) soya margarine 3 tablespoons olive oil 2 bay leaves	Melt together in a heavy pan until bubbling, then remove from the heat.
2 tablespoons organic white flour 1 tablespoon wholemeal (wholewheat) flour	Beat into melted fats to form a thick smooth paste.

600ml (1 pint/2½ cups) soya milk	Add slowly to the pan, beating well. Return to a gentle heat and stir until the sauce thickens. If lumps form, beat with a whisk until smooth. Allow to boil gently for 5 minutes.

1 tablespoon low-salt bouillon powder *2 tablespoons nutritional yeast flakes* *½ teaspoon grated nutmeg* *½ teaspoon ground black pepper*	Whisk into the sauce and remove from the heat.

2 tablespoons olive oil *2 cloves garlic, crushed* *1 medium marrow (vegetable marrow) peeled or* * unpeeled, deseeded and cut into approximately* * 10cm/4 inch slabs or large even rectangles*	Heat the oil in another heavy pan. Rub the garlic over the marrow pieces and turn each piece in the hot oil. Lower the heat, cover tightly and cook slowly for 5 minutes. Remove from the heat. Place half the marrow pieces in the bottom of a casserole or ovenproof dish. Cover with a good layer of bean sauce and then more marrow. Top with the creamy sauce and bake in the oven for 35–40 minutes until bubbling and golden on top. Don't fill the dish to the top as it does tend to overflow.

 This is a bit like a lighter form of lasagne but still satisfying and really tasty – a meal in itself with a salad. As with any lasagne it can be a bit time-consuming making all the layers first, so it is definitely worth cooking double or even triple the quantity of bean mixture and freezing it for the next time. Having some in the freezer will also be handy if you need a fast sauce for pasta.

For a change you can forget the layers. Just cut the marrow across into round slices about 4cm/1½ inches thick and scoop out the seeds. Place the slices on an oiled roasting tray and pile some bean sauce into the middle of each one. Cover with foil and bake at 180°C/350°F/Gas 4 for 35 minutes. Uncover and spoon some creamy sauce on top of each stuffed slice, then return to the oven for another 20 minutes until the marrow is really soft and the sauce is golden on top.

JAPANESE-STYLE KABOCHA STICKS WITH SESAME

750g/1½lb kabocha or Sweet Mama squash
2 tablespoons olive oil
2 teaspoons roasted sesame oil
150ml (5 fl oz/⅔ cup) water
1 teaspoon low-salt bouillon powder

Remove the seeds from the squash and cut into thin matchsticks (include the skin and use a strong sharp knife). Toss the oils and squash together over a high heat for 4 minutes. Add the water and bouillon powder, reduce the heat and cover tightly. Simmer for 10–15 minutes until the squash is soft and the liquid has been absorbed.

50g (2oz/½ cup) whole sesame seeds
1 tablespoon tamari soy sauce

Roast and toast the seeds in a dry frying pan for around 5 minutes, until they pop about and smell gorgeous. Grind briefly in a spice grinder or crush a little with a rolling pin and then sprinkle on top of the squash. Splash with the tamari and serve warm.

 When I have eaten this delicate dish in Japan the squash has been carefully cut into long, thin 'strings' and is often made with just the dark green skin with a tiny slither of the orange flesh lining it. It is very beautiful, but very time-consuming if you are not skilled with a scalpel. This is a faster version.

SUMMER SQUASH WITH LEEKS, PASTA AND ROASTED WALNUTS

4 medium courgettes (zucchini)
3 medium leeks, cleaned and sliced

Drop the whole courgettes (zucchini) and sliced leeks into a pan of boiling water and simmer for 10 minutes. Drain and leave to cool.

225g (8oz/2 cups) walnut pieces

Meanwhile, gently toast the walnuts in a heavy dry pan, shaking and stirring for about 5 minutes.

1 tablespoon cider vinegar or white wine vinegar
2 teaspoons balsamic vinegar
2 tablespoons grainy mustard, or mustard seeds soaked in vinegar and whizzed in a blender
1 teaspoon honey
2 tablespoons olive oil
1 tablespoon walnut oil
1 teaspoon ground black pepper
2 teaspoons tamari soy sauce – optional

Add the vinegar to the walnuts in the hot pan and let it sizzle madly for a couple of seconds. Remove from the heat and stir in the remaining ingredients.

225g (8oz/2⅔ cups) dried pasta shapes, cooked
handful of fresh parsley or basil, roughly chopped

Add to the pan. The courgettes (zucchini) should now be cool enough to handle, so slice them and add them along with the leeks. Mix thoroughly. Warm through to serve hot.

 Wholewheat and white pasta shells look pretty in this dish, which is lovely as it is or with a sauce of your choice. Served hot, it's nice with a creamed leak sauce; served warm, it's nice with tahini. It's also good cold with a vinaigrette dressing.

WINTER SQUASH AND SUNFLOWER RISOTTO

3 tablespoons olive oil

1 teaspoon dried thyme or 1 big sprig of
  fresh thyme

2 bay leaves

3 tablespoons sunflower seeds

Heat in a heavy pan for a few minutes to allow
the seeds to begin to toast.

1 onion, preferably red, finely chopped

Add to the pan, stir well and soften for 5
minutes.

450g/1lb winter squash, peeled, deseeded and cut
  into small bite-size pieces

½ teaspoon ground black pepper

2 good pinches of paprika

Stir into the onion and sizzle for 5 minutes.
Cover tightly, reduce the heat and cook for 10
minutes, stirring occasionally.

1 heaped teaspoon low-salt bouillon powder

1 good teaspoon low-salt yeast extract

2 teaspoons malt extract (malt syrup)

2 tablespoons organic red wine or red grape juice
  with a splash of cider vinegar

water to just cover

Add to the pan, stir well and bubble for 5
minutes. Continue to cook very gently for 10
minutes.

225g (8oz/1 cup) barley, cooked – see page 82

chopped fresh parsley

Stir the cooked barley into the pan, making
sure that everything is well mixed. Continue
to heat gently for 10 minutes. Serve sprinkled
with lots of fresh parsley.

An authentic risotto is made with Italian arborio rice, which has a certain springy, creamy, bite to it. Barley, although it has bigger grains, can still be used very successfully to get that real risotto texture. This dish is dark and similar to the earthy risotto of southern Italy.

Use any sweet-flavoured winter squash. Sometimes try replacing the seeds with pine kernels for a change of flavour.

A nice dark green salad goes well with this – try watercress or spinach and Cos lettuce. Also try a spoonful of Red Onion Relish (see page 25) on the side.

GINGERY WINTER SQUASH AND POTATO SOUP

---

2 tablespoons olive oil
5cm/2 inch piece of fresh root ginger, grated
2 bay leaves
2 medium potatoes, peeled and chopped
1 large onion, chopped

Heat the oil, ginger and bay leaves in a large heavy pan. Add the vegetables and cook gently until the onion begins to soften.

900g/2lb orange-fleshed winter squash or
   pumpkin, peeled, deseeded and chopped
900ml (1½ pints/3¾ cups) vegetable stock
   or water
2 teaspoons low-salt bouillon powder
juice of 2 oranges
grated zest (peel) of 1 orange
2 pinches of ground ginger

Add to the pan and simmer for 30 minutes until the potatoes are soft. Remove the bay leaves and whizz until smooth in a blender or food processor (you could also use a hand blender).

---

snipped fresh chives
black pepper

Reheat if necessary, then top with snipped chives and a grind or two of black pepper to serve.

THAMA'S VEGETABLE BHAJI

2 teaspoons whole cumin seeds

2 bay leaves

1 teaspoon black mustard seeds

1 teaspoon black onion seeds (kalonji/nigella)

2 small dried red chillies – optional

pinch of asafetida

6 tablespoons oil

1 large onion, thinly sliced

2.5cm/1 inch piece of fresh root ginger, grated

Heat the spices in the oil until just smoking and smelling nutty. Add the onion and ginger and stir well, then cook over a moderate heat until the onion is soft and beginning to brown.

---

1 level tablespoon turmeric

½ teaspoon chilli powder – optional

Sprinkle over the onion, stir and continue to cook for 3–4 minutes.

450g/1lb sweet pumpkin or winter squash, peeled, deseeded and cut into thin sticks – like thin fries

2 medium potatoes, unpeeled and cut in the same way – optional

1 medium courgette (zucchini), cut in the same way

Add to the pan and stir very well. Allow everything to sizzle and soften, cover, then reduce the heat and cook for 5 minutes.

---

3 tablespoons water

2 tablespoons tamari soy sauce

Splash over the vegetables and stir well, cover and continue to cook gently for 25 minutes. You will need to stir regularly and maybe add a few more splashes of water – you want to end up with the vegetables soft and browning but not burnt or stuck forever to the pan.

Some fresh coriander (cilantro) would be a nice final touch. Serve with rice or scoop up with Spinach Chapatis (see page 70).

Not only are my parents great cooks but my grandmother on my father's side taught us the wonderful skill of producing delicious dishes from apparently nothing at all, and I have adapted this from the one she used to make us for lunch by just using potatoes and onions. Thama is the Bengali word for paternal grandmother – it's what we all called her.

SIMPLY ROASTED WINTER SQUASH

OVEN: 220°C/425°F/GAS 7

750–900g/1½–2lb) orange-fleshed winter squash
2 tablespoons olive oil
2 cloves garlic, thinly sliced
1 tablespoon tamari soy sauce
pinch of ground black pepper

Remove the seeds from the squash and cut the flesh into thick slices or chunks. Toss everything in a large bowl and mix together to make sure that the squash is well coated. Turn into a big roasting tray so that the pieces are separate, or at least not too piled up. Bake in the oven for 35 minutes until soft and well browned in places.

This recipe will bring out the sweet delight of any of the winter squash varieties. I think it works best with kabocha or butternut. For ease I usually leave the skin on and deal with it on the plate – once it has been roasted it is often succulent and soft enough to eat, and it tastes delicious. If you are making this dish at the end of the season, or using an elderly squash, you may prefer to peel the skin off first.

Good as a side vegetable with almost anything, or try it warm on a bed of mixed salad leaves with a tiny splash of balsamic vinegar or lemon juice.

If you ever have any left over, it makes a great soup if whizzed up with soya milk, vegetable stock and fresh parsley.

STUFFED SQUASH

OVEN: 180C/350°F/GAS 4

4 small, 2 medium or 1 large squash

Remove the top by cutting in at an angle around the stem until you can remove the stem with a cone of flesh attached. Scoop out the seeds and strands and cut the cone of flesh from the stem to leave a little flat lid.

4 tablespoons olive oil (¼ cup)
4 bay leaves
2 teaspoons dried sage
1 teaspoon dried thyme
2 tablespoons sunflower seeds
2 medium onions, finely chopped
2 medium carrots, grated
any flesh from the squash 'lids', finely chopped

Heat the oil, add the leaves, herbs and seeds and sauté everything together over a gentle heat until soft, about 10 minutes.

2 fresh tomatoes, finely chopped
350g (12oz/1¾ cups) dried butter beans, rice or other grains, cooked
8 tablespoons (½ cup) water
2 teaspoons low-salt bouillon powder
½ teaspoon ground black pepper

Add to the pan and mix well. Cook over a gentle heat for about 10 minutes.

100g (4oz/2 cups) soft fresh wholemeal (wholewheat) breadcrumbs

Remove the pan from the heat and mash in the breadcrumbs to combine thoroughly. Pull out the bay leaves as they appear and rinse them off. You may need fewer breadcrumbs if you are using rice – the mix shouldn't be too dry.

Place the squash on a baking (cookie) tray, trimming the base of the squash a little if it does not stand up straight. Fill with the stuffing – don't pack it too tight. Replace the lids, tucking a bay leaf underneath, then bake in the oven for about 1 hour or until the flesh is soft but not collapsing. If the tops are browning too fast, just lay a sheet of foil on top.

Try serving with Gentle Onion Sauce (see page 23).

Sometimes it is just as good to bake the stuffing separately and serve it next to roasted or steamed squash. Go with how you feel on the day. This recipe is good for any squash, but I feel it can all get somewhat overwhelming if you use one of those giant orange pumpkins. If you've got lots of people to feed you may like to try, but double the stuffing and increase the cooking time if you do. Otherwise, choose patty pan, Sweet Mama, round butternut, Little Gem, kabocha or Delicata. If they are small, choose one per person or one between two.

PUMPKIN AND TOMATO BISQUE

1 large onion, chopped

6 tablespoons olive oil

2 teaspoons fresh or dried oregano leaves

1 teaspoon dulce pimienton, paprika or
   cayenne powder

Soften together over a moderate heat for 5 minutes.

---

1 tablespoon tomato paste

900g/2lb pumpkin or winter squash, peeled,
   deseeded and roughly chopped

1 small sweet red pepper (bell pepper),
   finely chopped

8 medium tomatoes, chopped

2 medium potatoes, chopped – optional

1 clove garlic, chopped

4 tablespoons low-salt bouillon powder

water

Let the tomato paste sizzle in with the onion for a couple of minutes and then add the vegetables, bouillon powder and water to cover well. Bring to the boil, reduce the heat and simmer covered for about 20 minutes, until the potatoes are soft.

300ml (10 fl oz/1⅓ cups) soya milk

½ teaspoon ground black pepper

½ teaspoon ground nutmeg

1 tablespoon tamari soy sauce – optional

Add to the pan, stir well and simmer for a further 10 minutes. Cool a little, then whizz until smooth in a blender or food processor (you could also use a hand blender). You should have smooth soup with a velvety texture, so add a little more soya milk if it is too thick.

 Garlic or pesto croûtons are nice scattered on the top to serve. To make them, just brush some toast with olive oil and spread with a little crushed garlic or some pesto, and grill (broil) or bake in the oven for a few minutes. Cut into little squares and use immediately.

It is worth searching for dulce pimienton powder for this recipe as it gives an interesting smoky flavour. Look in the spice shelves at the supermarket.

THIS BUSINESS
OF BEANS

For some, the idea of beans does not naturally excite thoughts of wondrous creative cookery, but this is very much an attitude of our modern society. The entire Asian world has prized, delighted in and depended upon this amazingly diverse source of goodness for over a thousand years.

The whole family of beans, peas and lentils are known collectively as legume vegetables – defined as plants whose edible seeds grow inside pods after the flowers die off. It is a truly enormous family, and a few of them that you are likely to encounter in your shopping are:

Aduki
Black beans
Black-eyed peas (beans)
Broad (fava) beans
Butter beans
Cannellini beans
Chick peas (garbanzo beans)
Flageolet beans
Green peas
Haricot (navy) beans
Kidney beans
Mung beans
Pinto beans
Soya beans

Lentils are various kinds of beans and peas that have had their outer skin removed and have been split in half during drying, so in general they contain a little less fibre and cook more quickly.

All beans can be eaten young and fresh in their pods or matured and dried for storing.

Beans and lentils are low in calories and fats and are an extremely good source of complex carbohydrates. Most importantly, they are a valuable source of protein in this approach to health. Sadly, it seems they are also the source of much confusion – do they supply enough? Is it in the right form for our bodies to use? Yes, is the answer to both questions in this way of eating, as the inclusion of whole grains and fresh vegetables in the diet ensures that all the amino acids (the building blocks of proteins) are readily available. Another concern with beans is that for some people they may increase gas in the digestive tract, causing flatulence and abdominal discomfort. If you do find that some beans have this effect on you, either try other kinds of beans, or soak them overnight before cooking to dissolve out some of the oligosaccharides (starch-like molecules) that can cause the gut to react in this way. Red kidney beans must *always* be soaked and rinsed, boiled for a full 10 minutes and rinsed again before cooking – for me, this is a strong case for using a can on the odd occasion that you fancy red kidney beans. Chewing them well helps reduce any digestive problems, as does making them into pâtés, sauces and purées.

Beans and lentils are real 'super foods', so a little and often is perhaps easier on the digestion than trying to base meals on them. Add a few to soups and casseroles, have bean pâté on toast or in sandwiches, throw a handful into salads. Having small portions of cooked beans in the freezer helps make this easier. Cooking them is also easy whether you soak them or not: wash them well and put them in a large pan, cover with cold water and boil gently until they are very soft. Big beans take longer than little beans to get soft, but you don't need to watch, stir or concentrate on any of them. They cook by themselves while you do something else.

If you do resort to canned beans sometimes, always check the label and try to avoid added salt, sugar and chemical preservatives.

As this chapter is about embracing the bean, I thought it would also be a suitable place to include tofu, an extraordinary product that is made from soya beans. Very low in fat and very high in protein, once you get the hang of it you will be amazed just how delicious tofu can be. I say amazed because I am well aware that many of you will have tried it once and abandoned the whole idea in horror. I cannot deny that I have been offered white, tasteless and slippery cubes under the guise of 'vegetarian dish' and, even with my open embrace of all things beanie, have found myself unable to see the point in suffering in this way.

Always keep your eye on the joy of life, especially where tofu is concerned. To give you a new approach I have included recipes here using frozen tofu, which has a much more satisfying and 'chewy' texture. Some of the most expensive and delicious tofu available in Japan (its ancestral home) is that which has been 'snow-dried' in sacred mountains. You can create your own sacred version in your freezer. I try to always keep some frozen, cut into cubes and strips, with or without garlic, ginger, herbs, ready for fast food or creative experiment. Freeze the pieces spread out on a tray, then pack loosely in bags so they don't stick together. Take out as much as you need, drop it into boiling water and boil until thawed (3–10 minutes depending on size), then drain and squeeze out the water. The more you squeeze out the more chewy or 'meaty' the result. Use for any of the recipes.

APPROXIMATE COOKING TIMES FOR BEANS

FOR 225G (8OZ/1 CUP) DRY WEIGHT IN 4 TIMES THE AMOUNT OF WATER

BEAN TYPE	SIMMERING TIME	COOKED YIELD
Aduki	1 hour	2 cups
Butter beans	3 hours	2 cups
Black-eyed peas (beans)	1 hour	2 cups
Chick peas (garbanzo beans)	3 hours	2 cups
Cannellini	2 hours	2 cups
Flageolets	1^1/$_2$ hours	2 cups
Pinto beans	2 hours	2 cups
Mung beans	30–35 minutes	2^1/$_2$ cups
Lentils (water varies)	35–40 minutes	2^1/$_4$ cups

Bear in mind that beans are notorious for not conforming exactly. Keep cooking until they are tender and soft

CREAMY BUTTER BEAN AND LEEK CRUMBLE

OVEN: 180°C/350°F/GAS 4

5 tablespoons olive oil
2 teaspoons dried sage
1 teaspoon dried thyme
6 medium leeks, washed and green part shredded,
white part cut into 2.5cm/1 inch rounds
1 tablespoon low-salt bouillon powder
1 teaspoon ground nutmeg
1 teaspoon ground black pepper

Heat the oil and herbs in heavy pan, then add the leeks and other ingredients with a good splash of water. Stir well and simmer for about 15 minutes until the leeks are soft. Pour into a sieve (strainer) or colander over a bowl to catch the juices.

1 kg (2lb/4 big cups) cooked butter beans
leek juices
juice of 1 lemon
2 tablespoons tamari soy sauce
soya milk

Put half of the cooked beans in a blender or food processor, then add the leek juices followed by the lemon juice and tamari. Pour in enough soya milk to cover the beans by about 2.5cm/1 inch – this will depend on how juicy your leeks were. Whizz to a thick, creamy sauce. Stir into the leeks and the rest of the beans, then spoon into an ovenproof dish.

6 tablespoons olive oil
225g (8oz/4 cups) soft wholemeal (wholewheat)
breadcrumbs or 100g (4oz/2 cups) breadcrumbs
and 100g (4oz/1 cup) chopped nuts
grated zest (peel) of 1 lemon
1 clove garlic, crushed
1 tablespoon nutritional yeast flakes – optional
1 tablespoon tamari soy sauce

Mix together thoroughly, sprinkle on top of the bean mixture and bake in the oven for 30 minutes.

 Enjoy with baked potatoes and a lemony tomato and cucumber salad.

CITRON BRAISED ARTICHOKES WITH WHITE BEANS

1 medium onion, thinly sliced *1 small lemon, deseeded and thinly sliced* *6 tablespoons olive oil* *1 tablespoon finely chopped fresh thyme leaves* *pinch of ground black pepper* *1 bay leaf* *10 whole cloves garlic*	Soften together in a big heavy pan for about 10 minutes.
16 baby artichokes, washed, spiky tops snipped off and stems trimmed. If they are bigger than an egg, cut in half	Increase the heat and add to the pan. Sizzle madly until the artichokes begin to brown a little.
white wine or vegetable stock or both, to cover	Add to the pan so that the artichokes are just covered. Bubble for 5 minutes. Continue to simmer gently, partially covered, for 15 minutes.
350g (12oz/2 cups) cooked white beans, such as cannellini, flageolets, lima or small butter (navy) beans	Add to the pan with a little of the liquid from cooking (or from the can if you are using canned beans). Cover and simmer for another 10 minutes.
juice of 1 lemon *handful of chopped fresh parsley*	Sprinkle on top and serve hot or cold.

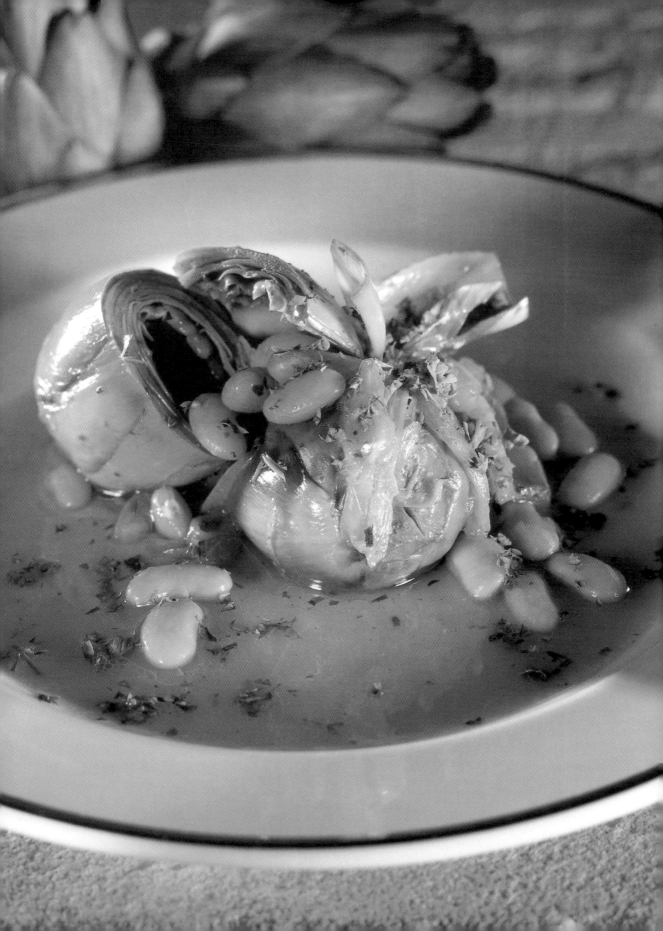

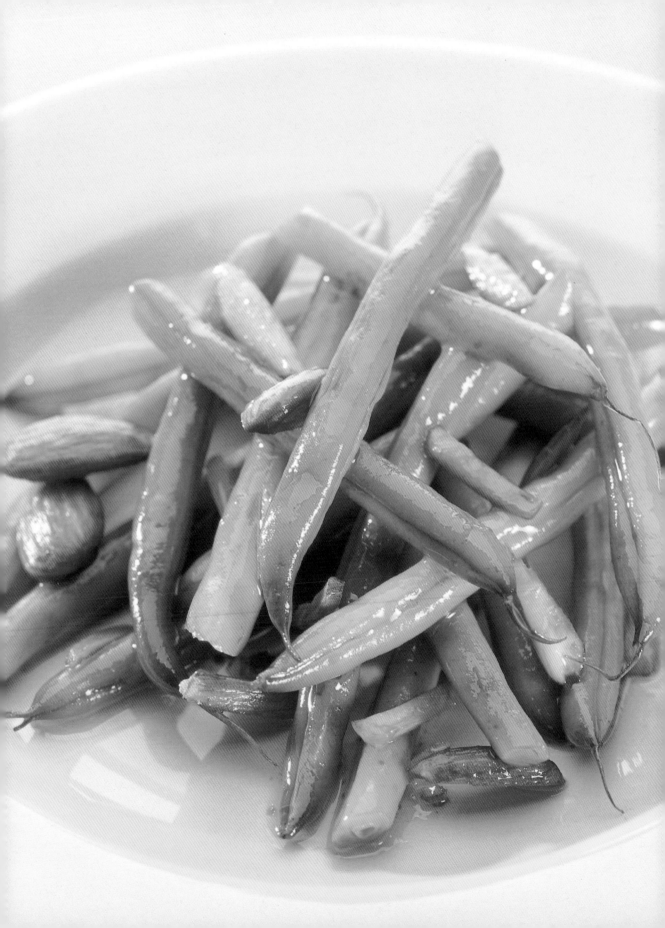

The perfect artichokes for this dish are the babies, which are about the size of an egg. Unfortunately, unless you grow them yourself, the chances of finding them are pretty limited. Farmers' markets and Italian suppliers are the most likely source. If you can't find them have a go with bigger ones, but they should be no bigger than a tennis ball and you will need only six. Wash them, cut off the top thirds with a sharp knife and trim the stems and one layer of leaves around the base. Cut each into four and trim out the hairy bits (the chokes) and the inner cones of leaves just above.

For a change, this recipe is also delicious using fresh, young broad (fava) beans instead of dried.

GREEN BEANS WITH GARLIC AND ALMONDS

450g/1lb French, green or bobby beans	Drop into boiling water and boil for 10 minutes. Drain and pile into a warm serving dish.
3 tablespoons olive oil *2 cloves garlic, thinly sliced* *100g (4oz/1 cup) slivered or whole almonds* *2 tablespoons tamari soy sauce*	Gently heat the oil with the garlic until it is just turning golden, quickly toss in the almonds and the tamari, stir and brown a few minutes longer. Tip over the green beans. Serve immediately.

 I have used fresh green beans in this recipe, but this mixture will liven up cooked dried beans too. Exchanging the almonds for other nuts or seeds makes combinations endlessly delicious, eg soft cooked butter beans and walnuts, or chick peas (garbanzo beans) with hazelnuts (filberts).

TOFU CACCIATORE

350g (12oz/2 cups) frozen tofu pieces (see page 135)
flour or polenta meal, for dusting
pinch of dried oregano
olive oil

Drop the tofu pieces, one by one, into boiling water. Boil for a few minutes, retrieve them with a slotted spoon and lay them on kitchen paper to drain. Dust with flour or polenta meal mixed with a pinch of oregano, then sauté them in a little olive oil until starting to brown. Set aside.

8 tablespoons (½ cup) olive oil
1 teaspoon dried oregano or a handful of fresh oregano
1 teaspoon dried basil
1 teaspoon ground black pepper
2 medium onions, finely chopped
4 cloves garlic, sliced
2 celery stalks, very finely chopped
1 carrot, grated

Heat the oil with the herbs and pepper and add everything else to the pan. Stir well over a moderate heat for 4–5 minutes. Reduce the heat, cover and cook until the vegetables are really soft and slushy.

4 tablespoons (¼ cup) tomato paste
8 good ripe tomatoes, chopped, or 2 x 400g/ 14oz cans
2 tablespoons malt extract (malt syrup)
1 teaspoon low-salt bouillon powder
1 tablespoon tamari soy sauce

Stir the tomato paste into the vegetables and stir-fry for 5 minutes. Add the other ingredients, stirring after each addition. Simmer very gently without the lid for 5 minutes. Drop in the pieces of tofu, add a little water or red wine if it is starting to stick and continue to simmer for 20 minutes.

 Cacciatore is a rich and delicious tomato sauce often served with chicken in Italy. It works well with tofu, and it's good served with spaghetti or buckwheat noodles and a green salad.

BEAN AND MUSHROOM PÂTÉ

2 teaspoons dried sage
1 teaspoon dried thyme
1 bay leaf
3 tablespoons olive oil
1 medium onion, very finely chopped
2 cloves garlic, chopped

Heat the herbs in the oil, add the onion and garlic and soften over a gentle heat for 8 minutes.

1 teaspoon tomato paste
350g (12oz/3 cups) mushrooms, chopped
1 teaspoon ground black pepper

Increase the heat, add the tomato paste and sizzle for a minute or two before adding the mushrooms and pepper. Mix well.

3 tablespoons tamari soy sauce
1 tablespoon water

Stir in the tamari and water, cover and lower the heat again. Allow to simmer very gently for 10 minutes.

350g (12oz/2 cups) cooked beans of your choice
olive oil, for drizzling

Pulse the beans in a blender or food processor, or mash to make a coarse purée. Add the mushroom mix, either stirring and mashing for a coarse-textured pâté, or whizzing in the blender or food processor for a smooth one. Press into a bowl, drizzle with olive oil and chill.

 This pâté looks pretty in little individual ramekin dishes for a first course. Serve with hot bread or thick toast. Keep some for lunchtime sandwiches.

Use whichever beans you have to hand or fancy at the time – mung beans seem to give a kind of liver pâté flavour, good served with lemon wedges. Kidney or aduki beans make it dark and rich, nice with orange wedges. Butter beans or cannellini make a creamy pâté, just crying out for a sprinkle of fresh parsley or chives.

BLACK AND RED CHILLI BEANS

225g (8oz/1⅓ cups) dried black beans or haricot
  (navy) beans
225g (8oz/heaping 1 cup) dried aduki beans

Bring to the boil in plenty of water and boil for 10 minutes. Switch off the heat and leave to stand for 10 minutes before draining. Return the beans to the clean pan and cover with fresh water. Bring to the boil and simmer for 1–1½ hours until the black beans are soft and the aduki beans are almost breaking up.

1 tablespoon malt extract (malt syrup)
6 fresh tomatoes, finely chopped
2 tablespoons low-salt bouillon powder
600ml (1 pint/2½ cups) water

Add to the beans, increase the heat and allow to bubble away gently to reduce the liquid – the beans will begin to break up and thicken it. Stir from time to time to stop everything sticking to the pan.

4 tablespoons (¼ cup) olive oil
2 teaspoons dried oregano
2 bay leaves
2 teaspoons whole cumin seeds
3 onions, chopped
10 cloves garlic, chopped
1 fresh red chilli, chopped

Heat the oil and the herbs and cumin seeds in another smaller pan. Add the onions, garlic and chilli and soften for about 5 minutes.

3 tablespoons tomato paste
1 tablespoon ground cumin
1 teaspoon paprika or pimienton dulce

Stir into the onions and cook for 5 minutes before adding the entire contents of the bean pan. Continue to gently simmer, uncovered, until thick and rich. The consistency shouldn't be soupy, but neither should it be so thick that it becomes solid and sticks to the pan.

Serve over rice or use to fill tortillas.

Try whizzing 100g (4oz/¹/₂ cup) plain silken tofu with the grated zest (peel) and juice of a lime, a splash of tamari and a pinch of black pepper to make a 'sour cream' topping.

This is a variation of an old favourite. In a few recipes, this one included, you will notice there is a little extra process at the beginning of bean cooking. This is because these dishes include the water that the beans have been cooked in and the flavour is better if you include the initial water change in the process. If you are using canned beans, rinse them and add fresh water.

A really good chilli takes time to develop and it is worth making this the day before you want to serve it. This recipe is generous and it freezes well.

HERB BRAISED LENTILS

450g (1lb/heaping 2 cups) whole lentils –
    brown, green or Puy
3 tablespoons olive oil
1 teaspoon low-salt bouillon powder
2 thick slices of lemon
4 cloves garlic, or as much as you like, cut in half
sprig or two of fresh thyme or 1 teaspoon
    dried thyme
sprig or two of fresh rosemary or 1 teaspoon
    dried rosemary
2 tablespoons apple juice
water

Cover with water and bring to the boil. Reduce the heat to a quiet simmer, cover and cook for 35–40 minutes until the lentils are soft but not breaking up. Increase the heat and reduce any remaining liquid to a juice of about 2.5cm/1 inch in the bottom of the lentils.

Have this with a cooked grain or with Roasted Marvels (see page 95). This is quite a generous amount for four to allow for leftovers, as the lentils are also very good cold or mixed into a green salad.

BUDAPEST BLACK-EYED PIE

OVEN: 200°C/400°F/GAS 6

*225g (8oz/1⅓ cups) dried black-eyed peas (beans),
    simmered for about 1 hour or until really soft*
*50g (2oz/⅓ cup) creamed coconut from a block,
    chopped*

Drain the beans and drop the coconut into the pan with them. Cover and leave to melt.

---

*175g (6oz/1 cup) oatmeal or 175g (6oz/2 cups)
    oats*
175g (6oz/1½ cups) sunflower seeds
3 tablespoons olive oil
2 teaspoons sesame oil – optional

Mix in a food processor with a sharp blade until the mixture resembles a coarse crumbly texture. Reserve about one-third of the mix and press the rest into the bottom of an oiled quiche pan (about 25cm/10 inch round, preferably with a loose base). Place in the oven for 10 minutes. Keep an eye on it and take it out when it's just browning.

---

4 tablespoons (¼ cup) olive oil
3 medium onions, finely chopped
4 cloves garlic, finely chopped

Soften together gently for 10 minutes or so until the onions are really soft.

---

2 tablespoons tomato paste
2 teaspoons paprika
2 teaspoons low-salt yeast extract
½ teaspoon ground black pepper
2 teaspoons cider vinegar or lemon juice

Stir into the onions and sizzle for a few minutes. Tip in the beans and coconut and mash to mix well. Pile the mixture into the quiche pan, flatten gently and sprinkle the remaining sunflower mix on the top. Give it a little pat down and bake in the oven at 190°C/375°F/Gas 5 for 15–20 minutes. Let it stand for 10 minutes before serving warm.

 This is also very good cold. Try it with baked potatoes, green salad and a rootsie rémoulade.

MIDDLE EASTERN BEAN AND VEGETABLE CASSEROLE

225g (8oz/heaping 1 cup) dried beans, such as haricots (navy), cannellini or flageolets

Bring to the boil in a large pan of water, boil for 10 minutes and remove from the heat. Allow to stand for 10 minutes, then drain. Return the beans to the cleaned pan, add 5 cups water and bring to the boil. Simmer for approximately 1½ hours.

1 large onion, chopped
225g (8oz/1⅔ cups) celeriac (celery root), peeled and chopped
1 medium carrot, scrubbed or peeled and chopped
5 tomatoes, chopped
4 cloves garlic, sliced
handful of fresh parsley, chopped
sprigs or sprinklings of fresh or dried thyme, rosemary and oregano
1 tablespoon low-salt bouillon powder
½ teaspoon ground black pepper
1 teaspoon ground cumin

Add to the beans and their liquid, cover and continue to simmer gently for 45 minutes until the beans are very soft. If you want to go away and do something else, it is best to do this in the oven at 180°C/350°F/Gas 4.

juice of 1 lemon
2 tablespoons olive oil – optional
handful of fresh parsley, roughly chopped

Stir into the beans, squashing some of them against the side of the pan with a spoon to thicken the juices.

 Another one-pot wonder, but not one to try and hurry. Serve in wide shallow bowls with bread, or with toast spread with Triple Tomato Pesto (see page 94).

BULGAR WHEAT WITH BEANS AND CUMIN

225g (8oz/1 cup) mung beans	Cook in simmering water for 30–35 minutes until soft. Drain.
250g (10oz/heaping 1½ cups) bulgar wheat *2 teaspoons low-salt bouillon powder*	Cover in boiling water and leave to stand for 30 minutes. All the water should be absorbed and the grain tender and fluffy. If there is more than a trace of water at the bottom of the bowl, just drain it off.
1 tablespoon cumin seeds *2 bay leaves* *4 tablespoons (¼ cup) olive oil* *2 medium onions, finely chopped*	Roast the seeds and bay leaves in the oil until well browned. Add the onions and stir well for a few minutes. Lower the heat, and soften the onions for 5 minutes.
1 teaspoon ground cumin *1 teaspoon paprika* *1 teaspoon ground black pepper* *1 tablespoon tamari soy sauce – optional* *juice of 1 lemon*	Stir into the onions and sizzle for a bit.
225g (8oz/heaping 1 cup) cooked broad (fava) *beans – frozen are fine if fresh are not in season*	Stir into the onions with the bulgar and mung beans. Just heat through to serve.

 This is another dish which is endlessly versatile. Once you've got the hang of it, experiment with other grains and combinations of beans. I love it sprinkled with fresh coriander (cilantro), lemon zest (peel) and fresh green chillies.

SWEET AND UNREFINED LIFE

Sugar is a refined form of carbohydrate, and it is one of the forms of carbohydrate to avoid. We have become extremely accustomed to the sweet treats in life and often add to our sugar load unknowingly when we eat packaged and processed foods.

Because we have become accustomed to these flavours in our food and often want to be able to serve them to friends and family, I have included them in this book, but I feel I would just like to remind you that although forms and effects vary, anything described as syrup or honey is sugar. The benefit of using forms other than the refined crystals is really in the speed with which they enter our bloodstream. Being carbohydrates means they are providers of energy, the problem is that whereas complex carbohydrates such as grains and whole foods provide a slow release of energy over a sustained period, simple carbohydrates like sugars are the equivalent of high-octane aviation fluid. This puts our systems into overdrive, is wasteful of other nutrients and leads to what could be described as metabolic overdraft – we go into energy debt and use up lots trying to constantly repay it – as with all overdrafts it's a pretty vicious cycle. We are aiming at keeping blood sugar levels stable without highs and lows and consequent energy drain. Sugar is calories without nutrients. Natural fruit syrups, concentrates and honeys are forms of sugar but with some nutrients.

What all this means is that for best health you should eat a lot of whole foods and occasionally choose to use forms of sweetness that are not in crystals. Fresh and dried fruits are the very best ways of doing this, so sometimes try some of the scrummy recipes in this chapter.

SPICE AND FRUIT CAKE

OVEN: 180°C/350°F/GAS 4

225g (8oz/1½ cups) sultanas (golden raisins)

100g (4oz/¾ cup) soaked fruit, such as apricots, prunes and/or figs

2 tablespoons malt extract (malt syrup)

2 tablespoons date syrup

2 tablespoons honey

225ml (7½ fl oz/scant 1 cup) apple juice

Melt together in a pan and remove from the heat.

225g (8oz/1½ cups) organic white flour

225g (8oz/1½ cups) wholemeal (wholewheat) flour

4 teaspoons baking powder

1 tablespoon ground mixed spice (apple pie spice)

100g (4oz/½ cup) soya margarine

Sift the dry ingredients into a large mixing bowl and rub in the fat as for pastry until the mixture resembles rough breadcrumbs.

Quickly stir in the melted mixture and turn into a greased 25cm/10 inch round cake pan or 1 kg/2lb loaf pan. Bake in the oven for 1¼ hours.

 A really reliable, basic fruit cake that freezes well. It has lots of vitamins and it will give you enough energy to climb mountains.

APPLE COMPOTE WITH ALMOND CREAM TOPPING

6 Cox's or other sweet apples, cored and roughly
    chopped
3 tablespoons lemon juice
2 tablespoons apple juice

Bring to the boil over a moderate heat, stir and cover tightly, then reduce the heat and simmer gently for 25 minutes. If it starts to catch, add a splash more apple juice. Cool a little and whizz to a smooth purée in a food processor or blender. Divide between individual serving glasses.

175g (6oz/heaping 1 cup) almonds
300ml (10 fl oz/1¼ cups) apple juice or half soya
    and half apple juice
½ teaspoon almond extract

Whizz the almonds to a fine powder in the food processor or blender. If they are reluctant, switch the machine off and give the whole thing a good shake. Whizz again and repeat a couple of times. Slowly add the liquid until you have the desired consistency, which should be like single (light) cream. Whizz in the almond extract. Use as a topping for the apples. Chill to serve.

 This is a really simple and gorgeous dessert that looks very smart in glasses with a dusting of ground cinnamon or a topping of some crunchy Honey Caramelized Almonds (see page 151). I think it is well worth keeping a bowl of apple purée in the fridge for those day-to-day needs when you want a spoonful of something soothing.

SPICED APPLE CAKE

OVEN: 180°C/350°F/GAS 4

450g/1lb sweet apples, grated with skin on
475ml (16 fl oz/2 cups) boiling water
300g (10 oz/2 cups) raisins
3 tablespoons olive oil
150g (5oz/scant ½ cup) honey
2 tablespoons maple syrup
2 teaspoons ground cinnamon
2 teaspoons ground nutmeg
½ teaspoon ground cloves

Mix together in a large bowl and leave to cool a little.

450g (1lb/heaping 3 cups) wholemeal
  (wholewheat) flour
2 teaspoons baking powder

Sift together into the bowl and mix in quickly. Turn into a greased 25cm/10 inch round cake pan or 1 kg/2lb loaf pan and bake in the oven for 1 hour. Test with a skewer – if it comes out a bit sticky, allow another 10 minutes cooking time. Cool, wrap tightly and store in an airtight container.

A moist cake that keeps really well – as long as no-one knows where it is.

HONEY CARAMELIZED ALMONDS

225g (8oz/1½ cups) whole almonds
8 tablespoons runny honey

Toast the almonds in a heavy frying pan. When they begin to brown and smell heavenly, carefully pour in the honey. Stir well but take care as the honey will bubble like mad and can burn easily. When the almonds are coated and the honey is dark golden brown, tip on to a sheet of non-stick parchment paper and cool. Use them whole, chopped or completely crushed to a fine praline powder.

Sprinklings of this delicious treat make a good topping or decoration for desserts. They will transform your morning cereal or porridge. Once cool, keep them in an airtight jar or they will go soft. This recipe uses almonds, but it will work well with other nuts or mixtures of nuts.

DO-IT-YOURSELF VITAMIN AND MINERAL SUPPLEMENTS

2 teaspoons linseed (flaxseed)
100g (4oz/¼ cup) pumpkin seeds
100g (4oz/¼ cup) sesame seeds
100g (4oz/¼ cup) sunflower seeds
175g (6oz/scant 1 cup) unsulphured dried apricots
50g (2oz/⅓ cup) any other dried fruit such as
  plump raisins, currants, prunes, dates or figs
sesame seeds, carob powder or desiccated
  (shredded) coconut, for coating

Mix to a pulp in a food processor with a sharp blade. If you find the linseeds stay whole for the first time you try this, it may be worth grinding the seeds separately first as they can be quite chewy.

Take heaped teaspoons of the mixture and roll in sesame seeds, carob powder or coconut. This should make about 30 little balls.

 If you have some small paper confectionery (candy) cases you can just press a spoonful of the mixture into them and not bother with the coating and rolling part.

You can vary the flavour as you choose with cardamom seeds, ground nuts, ground ginger or cinnamon, or with vanilla extract.

Refrigerate and eat regularly.

Probably the biggest vitamin tablets in the world. Don't worry that they don't taste remotely like medicine – they are scrumptious and kids love them too. They are a great addition to packed lunches or eaten as a snack.

One of these little wonders a day will supply many necessary vitamins and minerals. They are particularly rich in potassium and calcium.

DATE AND MALT TEA LOAF

OVEN: 190°C/375°F/GAS 5

*600ml (1 pint/2½ cups) weak tea – Earl Grey
   is nice*
450g (1lb/3 cups) pitted dates

Simmer gently for approximately 20 minutes until the dates are soft. Mash to absorb the liquid.

225g (8oz/1 cup) malt extract (malt syrup)
2 tablespoons date syrup

Add to the date mixture and allow to cool a little.

225g (8oz/1½ cups) wholemeal (wholewheat) flour
100g (4oz/scant 1 cup) organic white flour
1 teaspoon ground ginger
1 teaspoon ground nutmeg
1 teaspoon ground mixed spice (apple pie spice)

Sift into a large bowl and quickly and thoroughly stir into the date mixture. Turn into a greased and lined 900g/2lb loaf pan and bake in the oven for 40 minutes. Lower the heat and continue cooking for a further 20 minutes. Cool in the pan, remove and wrap tightly. Store overnight before slicing to serve.

 Sticky and tasty. It gets better and better on keeping.

AROMATIC BRAISED APRICOTS

6 cardamom pods
450g/1lb unsulphured dried apricots
5cm/2 inch stick of cinnamon
water to cover

Press the cardamom pods gently with the back of a spoon to split them open. Put everything in a saucepan with a tight lid and bring to the boil. Simmer very, very gently until the fruits are soft and the liquor rich – this should take 30–40 minutes.

They are lovely served warm or cold, with Vanilla Pannacotta (see page 157).

If you have the oven on for something else, these do just as well baked.

CASHEW CREAM

225g (8oz/1½ cups) plain cashew nuts, broken
    pieces are fine
450ml (15 fl oz/scant 2 cups) apple juice

Put the nuts into a blender or food processor and whizz to a fine powder – you may need to stop and start a few times to give them a shake. The finer the powder the smoother the cream. Add the apple juice slowly with the machine on its slowest setting. You will end up with a thick cream, which you can then adapt to the consistency you want by adding more apple juice and/or soya milk.

When you are in the mood for cream but are avoiding dairy foods, this is the answer.

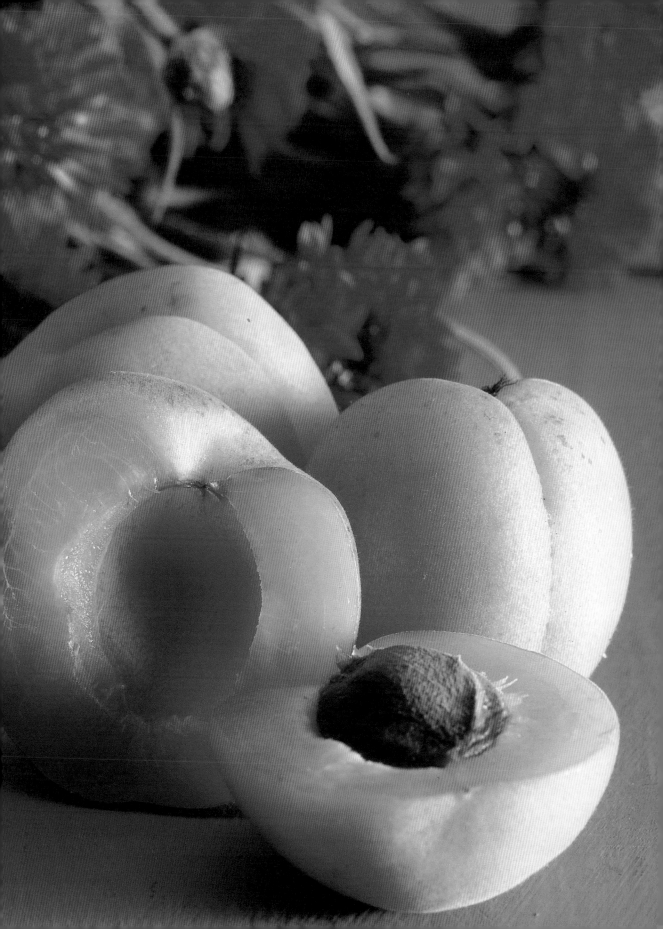

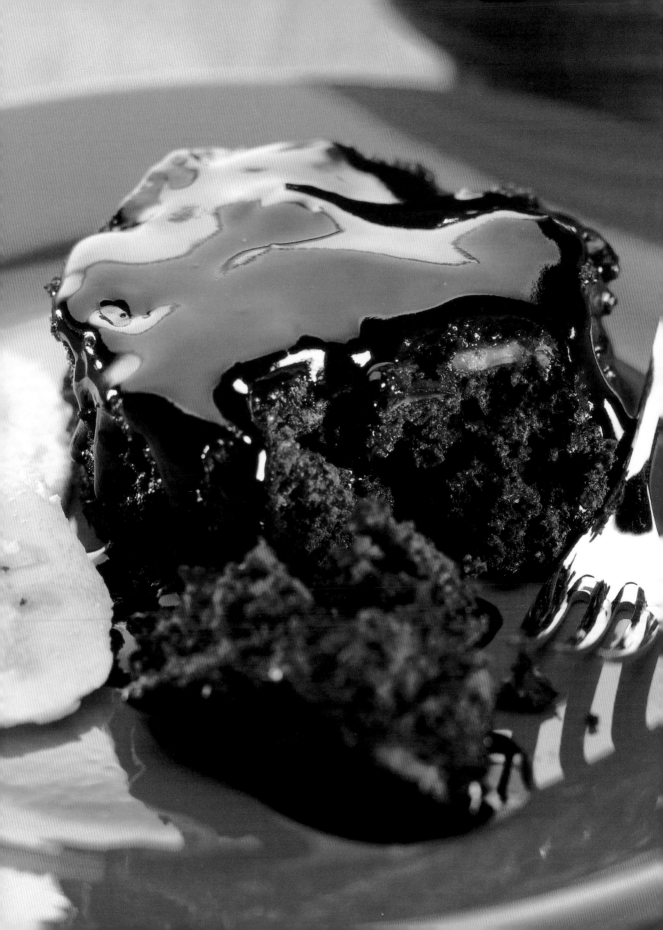

STICKY 'NOT CHOCOLATE' AND BANANA PUDDING

OVEN: 180°C/350°F/GAS 4

6 tablespoons malt extract (malt syrup) 6 tablespoons date syrup 300ml (10 fl oz/1¼ cups) apple juice 6 tablespoons carob powder 2 teaspoons vanilla extract	Melt together over a gentle heat, stirring until completely smooth. Bring to a gentle boil and stir for a few minutes more.
225g (8oz/1½ cups) wholemeal (wholewheat) flour 225g (8oz/1½ cups) organic white flour 1 tablespoon baking powder 175g (6oz/⅔ cup) soya margarine	Sift the dry ingredients into a bowl and rub in the margarine as for pastry until the mixture resembles rough breadcrumbs.
3 bananas, thinly sliced handful of carob drops – optional	Toss into the bowl and quickly stir in half of the carob sauce. Stir well to a soft dropping consistency. Turn into a greased ovenproof dish, pour the remaining sauce on top and gently splash with 4 tablespoons (¼ cup) warm water. Bake in the oven for 35–40 minutes.

 The top should be quite crunchy and the pudding should have a gooey sauce at the bottom of the dish.

JELLY WITHOUT GELATINE

1 heaped tablespoon agar agar flakes – if you have powder, use the quantity on the packet needed to set 600ml (1 pint/2½ cups)
200ml (7 fl oz/scant 1 cup) water

Heat together in a small saucepan and allow to boil for 4–5 minutes, whisking well as the mixture boils and froths. Whisk into …

200ml (7 fl oz/scant 1 cup) each natural fruit syrup and water or
400ml (14 fl oz/scant 2 cups) juiced fresh fruits such as strawberries and/or fresh oranges with a splash of fruit syrup

Mix together, then whisk in the agar agar mixture.

 Pour into a bowl or glasses to set, with or without a few pieces of fresh fruit. Agar, unlike gelatine, will set quickly at room temperature.

I could easily have included this in the chapter on sea vegetables, because agar agar is a nutrient derived from different forms of seaweed. It is invaluable as a setting agent when you do not want to use gelatine that is derived from the bones of animals, and it has no flavour – I promise that you will not feel you are eating seaweed. Let it reassure you of the diversity of the possibilities of sea vegetables if you are feeling a little unsure of trying any of my savoury recipes.

VANILLA PANNACOTTA

2 vanilla pods (beans)
600ml (1 pint/2½ cups) soya milk
2 teaspoons maple syrup

Split the vanilla pods lengthways, scrape out the seeds and add both the pods (beans) and the seeds to a heavy pan with half of the soya milk and all of the maple syrup. Heat gently for 20 minutes to infuse the flavours.

1 really heaped tablespoon agar agar flakes
8 tablespoons (½ cup) water

Bring to a furious boil in a separate small pan, whisk and boil for 4–5 minutes. Immediately whisk into the warm soya milk mixture, followed by the rest of the cold soya milk. Mix well, pour into 6 little moulds and chill. Turn out to serve with compotes or fruit purées.

 The original Italian classic is very rich with double (heavy) cream, but this light, low-fat version works well and looks lovely next to bright fruit.

FROZEN FRUIT CRUSH

fresh juice of 4 big oranges
finely grated zest (peel) of 2 oranges
300g (10oz/2½ cups) fresh strawberries or
   raspberries, cleaned
4 tablespoons (¼ cup) maple syrup

Whizz together in a blender or food processor. Pour into a shallow dish and freeze for 2–3 hours.

   Break into chunks and process again using a sharp blade until smooth and creamy. Return to the freezer for 30 minutes before serving. If you leave the fruit crush in the freezer for longer, leave it at room temperature for 45 minutes before serving, or until scoopable.

 For a change, try adding the following at the final whizz stage: 100g (4oz/½ cup) plain silken tofu, an extra 2 tablespoons maple syrup and 2 teaspoons vanilla extract.

If you have little ice-lolly moulds (popsicle molds), just leave the fruit crush longer at the final freeze and get them out when the sun is shining.

HEALTHY STORE CUPBOARD

A quick checklist to help you with your new style of shopping.

NUTS AND SEEDS

alfalfa seeds – for sprouting

almonds

Brazil nuts

cashew nuts

hazelnuts (filberts)

pine kernels

poppy seeds

pumpkin seeds

sesame seeds

sunflower seeds

walnuts

white poppy seeds – for availability try Asian stores

DRIED FRUITS

apricots – unsulphered

currants

dates

figs

prunes

raisins

sultanas (golden raisins)

DRIED HERBS

basil
bay leaves
mint
oregano
sage
tarragon
thyme
chives, parsley and coriander (cilantro) are best fresh

SPICES

asafetida – for availability try Asian stores
cardamom pods
cayenne pepper
cinnamon sticks
cloves
dulce pimienton
ground cinnamon
ground coriander
ground cumin
nutmeg
star anise
turmeric
whole coriander seeds
whole cumin seeds
whole yellow/black mustard seeds

OTHER FLAVOURINGS

agar agar flakes

almond extract

cider vinegar

low-salt bouillon powder

low-salt yeast spread

malt extract (malt syrup)

miso paste

nutritional yeast flakes

silken tofu

soya milk

tahini (sesame paste)

tamari soy sauce

tomato paste

vanilla extract

vanilla pod (bean)

FATS AND OILS

cold-pressed nut and seed oils

cold-pressed olive oil

cold-pressed sunflower oil

vegan soya margarine

GRAINS

barley

buckwheat

bulgar wheat

couscous

millet

oats

quinoa

rice – brown basmati, organic white basmati and whole brown

wheat berries (grain)

wild rice

PULSES (LEGUMES) AND PASTA

aduki beans
black-eyed peas (beans)
black beans
butter beans
cannellini beans
chick peas (garbanzo beans)
flageolets
haricot (navy) beans
lentils – brown, green, Puy and red
mung beans
pasta – rice, millet or buckwheat pasta and wholewheat pasta shapes
yellow split peas

SWEET FLAVOURINGS

apple juice concentrate
carob powder
date syrup
honey
maple syrup
organic apple juice
organic fruit concentrates
soya milk

FLOURS

100% wholewheat flour
brown rice flour
maize meal
organic white flour
polenta
soya flour

INDEX

broccoli 43
  broccoli pasta Arrabiata 46
  broccoli and potatoes with
    sesame and arame 60
  orange blasted broccoli 53
bronchitis 17
Brussels sprouts with nuts
  and lime 71
buckwheat 81, 82
Budapest black-eyed pie 144
bulbs 11, 17–19
bulgar wheat 82
  bulgar wheat with beans
    and cumin 146
butternut squash 120

cabbage
  ginger braised 79
  Kerala-style spiced 74
cakes
  spice and fruit 148
  spiced apple 150
calabrese 43
calcium 4, 67
cancer 1–2, 7, 90
carbohydrates 6, 30, 54
  complex 80, 134, 147
  refined 147
cardiovascular disease 17
carrots 30
  braised roots 39
  my Mum's perfect carrots 41
  winter veggie tarte tatin
    32–3
cashew cream 154
casseroles 134
  Middle Eastern bean and
    vegetable 145

cauliflower 43
  cauliflower braised in spicy
    cream 48–9
  cauliflower cheese without
    cheese 52–3
  minted cauliflower pureé
    51
celeriac 17
  creamed céléri-rave 21
celery root 17
  creamed céléri-rave 21
channa dhal with leaves 75
chick peas 18
Chinese leaves with miso
  dressing 118
chlorophyll 67
cholesterol 17, 90
chop suey 72–3
circulatory system 17
citron braised artichokes with
  white beans 138
cooking times
  beans 136
  grains 82
corn 80–1
  Tuscan polenta 103
courgettes 91, 119
  garlic rice galette 121
couscous 80, 82
creamy dishes
  butter bean and leek
    crumble 137
  céléri-rave 21
  garlic dip/sauce/soup 100
  onion gratin of dark green
    leaves 76
  vegetable risotto 102
crookneck 119

cucumber 119
    cucumber in creamy mint
        dressing 109
curiously green quiche 78

dairy free dauphinois 37
dairy produce 4, 5, 67
date and malt tea loaf 153
deficiencies 2, 67
digestion 8, 43, 134
dip, creamed garlic 100
do-it-yourself vitamin and
        mineral supplements 152
dressings 106
    black olive 92
    citrus 19
    creamy mint 109
    miso 118
dulse 55

eggplants 90
    herb and mustard roasted
        eggplant and potato 99
eggs 4
enzymes 18
equipment 8–9
essential fatty acids 8

fat 1, 5, 106, 134, 161
fennel 17
fibre 91, 119
fish 4, 5
flavourings 161, 162
flours 162
freezing 9
fresh mango salsa 110
frisson of frisée 108
frozen fruit crush 158

fruit 3, 6, 105, 106, 148, 159
    frozen fruit crush 158
    jelly without gelatine 156
    lavish fruit salad 107
fun, fire and delight 22

garbanzo beans 18
garlic 17, 90
    garlic rice galette 121
    garlic soup 23
gentle onion sauce 23
giant radish rémoulade 111
ginger
    ginger braised cabbage 79
    ginger brown rice and
        lentils 84
    gingery winter squash and
        potato soup 127
globe artichokes 43
    artichokes with mustard
        seed vinaigrette 44
    citron braised artichokes
        with white beans 138
gluten 81
golden nugget squash 119
golden tofu paella 102
gout 17
grains 3, 6, 14, 80–1, 134,
    161
    multiseed bread 85
gratin of roots with a twist 42
green beans with garlic and
    almonds 139
green caper relish 50

heart disease 7, 90
herbs 160
    herb braised lentils 143

These fabulous foods might just save your life. The follow up to Jane Sen's bestselling *Healing Foods Cookbook* is as delicious as healthy eating gets.

JANE SEN, winner of the BBC Radio 4 Award for Contributions to Healthy Eating, and Dietary Advisor to the renowned Bristol Cancer Help Centre, has produced a cookbook that feeds us on many levels. Her enthusiasm for cookery and simple delight in the ingredients is refreshing in a world where healthy eating all too often means foregoing the enjoyment of food.

These taste-filled, high-nutrition recipes, each free from meat, dairy and added salt or sugar, will boost your health and do you good - especially if your concerns include:

• Weight Loss • Digestive Problems • Heart Disease • Cancer
• Diabetes • Lack of Energy • Fertility Problems • Menopause

. . . .

PRAISE FOR JANE SEN'S *HEALING FOODS COOKBOOK*:

'...within a week I could feel the difference. I felt better and had a lot more energy.'
EXPRESS

'Exciting and unusual flavours - delicious enough to fob off to teenagers and children without their suspecting they are eating healthily. I recommend it.'
DEIRDRE MCQUILLAN, SUNDAY TELEGRAPH

'Sen's work, which revolves around a vegan, low-fat, -salt and -sugar diet has been recognized by hear disease charities for its contribution to healthy eating, and has inspired many cancer patients.'
SONIA PURNELL, GUARDIAN

. . . .

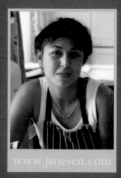

www.janesen.com

JANE SEN has worked with chefs throughout the world. She now lives near Bath and, as well as working as Dietary Advisor to the Bristol Cancer Help Centre, she cooks, writes and lectures all over the UK.

www.thorsons.com

UK £12.99*
US $19.95

ISBN 0-00-711834-1

*recommended price

9 780007 118342

Thorsons
Directions for Life

Cover photograph © Sian Irvine/The Anthony Blake Photo Library